Advances in Geriatric Dermatology

Anne Lynn S. Chang

Editor

Advances in Geriatric Dermatology

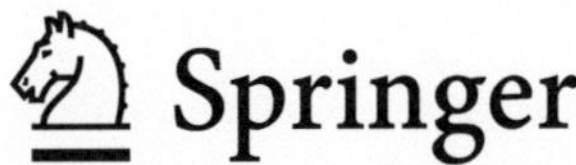 Springer

Editor
Anne Lynn S. Chang, MD
Assistant Professor of Dermatology
Standford University School of Medicine
Redwood City, CA, USA

ISBN 978-3-319-38725-3   ISBN 978-3-319-18380-0   (eBook)
DOI 10.1007/978-3-319-18380-0

Springer Cham Heidelberg New York Dordrecht London
© Springer International Publishing Switzerland 2015
Softcover reprint of the hardcover 1st edition 2015

Printed on acid-free paper

Springer International Publishing AG Switzerland is part of Springer Science+Business Media
(www.springer.com)

This book is dedicated to my colleagues who have a shared interest in medical issues of aging skin. Without their support, enthusiasm, dialogue, and thoughtful input, this work would not be possible.

Preface

This book is intended to synthesize current medical literature on critical topics in geriatric dermatology, a field that is likely to become more important as longevity in much of the world population increases. Historically, much of the field of skin aging has focused on aesthetics, but my career goal is to try to bridge the divide between the cosmetic aspects of skin aging and the very real medical issues of aging skin. Hopefully, this book will inspire other dermatologists as well as other physicians, researchers, and students to recognize the importance of medical issues of aging as it pertains to the skin. The ultimate goal is to spark research into these issues and narrow gaps in geriatric dermatology knowledge to improve patient care.

Redwood City, CA, USA   Anne Lynn S. Chang, MD

Acknowledgements

I wish to thank Maureen Alexander for her assistance in making this book a reality.

Contents

Contributors

Nason Azizi, M.D. Department of Dermatology, Stanford University School of Medicine, Redwood City, CA, USA

Staci Brandt, PA-C, M.B.A., M.S. Corporate Medical Affairs, Galderma Spirig, Egerkingen, Switzerland

Daniel C. Butler, M.D. Department of Dermatology, Massachusetts General Hospital, Boston, MA, USA

Anne Lynn S. Chang, M.D. Department of Dermatology, Stanford University School of Medicine, Redwood City, CA, USA

Gregory W. Charville Departments of Dermatology and Pathology, Stanford University School of Medicine, Redwood City, CA, USA

Justin Endo, M.D. Department of Dermatology, University of Wisconsin-Madison, Madison, WI, USA

Shannon Famenini, M.D. David Getier School of Medicine, Los Angeles, CA, USA

John Y.M. Koo, M.D. Department of Dermatology, UCSF, San Francisco, CA, USA

Olivia Yu-Ping Lai, B.S. Keck School of Medicine of the University of Southern California, School of Medicine, Los Angeles, CA, USA

Andy Liu, B.S. Albert Einstein College of Medicine, Bronx, NY, USA

Matthew Meckfessel, Ph.D. Medical Communications, Fort Worth, TX, USA

Robert A. Norman, D.O., M.P.H., M.B.A. University of Central Florida, College of Medicine, Tampa, FL, USA

Kevin Chun-Kai Wang, M.D., Ph.D. Department of Dermatology, Stanford University School of Medicine, Stanford, CA, USA

John Montgomery Yost, M.D., M.P.H. Department of Dermatology, Stanford University School of Medicine, Redwood City, CA, USA

Dermato-pharmacology in Older Patients

Olivia Yu-Ping Lai and Justin Endo

Physiologic Principles of Geropharmacology

Providers who treat older adult dermatology patients may hold preconceived notions—whether positive or negative—about the aging process and providing caring for this population. However, if one thinks of the characteristics of various older adult dermatology patients, a diversity of aging is likely to be found. The 90-year-old healthy, community-dwelling great-grandmother requesting a general skin check and refill of topical rosacea medications will be approached differently than the 70-year-old frail, institutionalized male with a non-operable basal cell carcinoma, unintentional weight loss, low performance status, poorly controlled psoriasis, and infected decubitus ulcers wishing to have aggressive therapy for all his conditions.

Aging is a heterogeneous process that results from an accumulation of both natural cellular senescence (i.e., "healthy" or intrinsic aging) and external factors (e.g., comorbid conditions, lifestyle, medications, environmental exposures) [1, 2]. As a result, older adults metabolize and respond differently to medications than younger adults. This fact might account for why older adults are four times more likely to be hospitalized for untoward drug events, over two-thirds of which are probably preventable [3]. Furthermore, it might not be possible to predict based solely on age how geriatric patients will respond to drugs. Age-related physiologic changes that are germane to the prescribing practitioner, or "geropharmacology," are highlighted, and the discussion focuses on pharmacokinetic (i.e., absorption, distribution, metabolism, and elimination of medications) and pharmacodynamic changes (i.e., the physiological effects of medications) [4]. In a later section, practical correlates of these geropharmacologic principles are demonstrated through common examples.

Pharmacokinetics of Aging

Medication Absorption

The two primary routes of dermatologic medication absorption are oral and topical. In healthy older adults, gastrointestinal (GI) and transdermal absorption do not appear to be significantly decreased compared to younger patients, despite changes in GI motility and age-related epidermal atrophy, respectively [5, 6]. Obviously, some older patients might have other comorbidities

O.Y.-P. Lai, B.S.
Keck School of Medicine of the University
of Southern California, Health Sciences Campus,
1975 Zonal Avenue, Los Angeles, CA 90089, USA
e-mail: olai@usc.edu

J. Endo, M.D. (✉)
Clinical Assistant Professor, Department of
Dermatology, University of Wisconsin-Madison,
1 South Park Street, 7th Floor,
Madison, WI 53715, USA
e-mail: jendo@dermatology.wisc.edu

© Springer International Publishing Switzerland 2015
A.L.S. Chang (ed.), *Advances in Geriatric Dermatology*, DOI 10.1007/978-3-319-18380-0_1

or surgeries that affect medication absorption. Therefore, the alterations in medication absorption should be taken into consideration when prescribing to these patients.

Volume of Distribution

The volume of distribution (Vd) is a theoretical construct that relates the amount of medication in the body (extravascular space) with respect to the medication's concentration in the blood or plasma [4]. Vd is not only affected by a given medication's chemical properties, but also by two primary physiologic characteristics that tend to change with aging: plasma proteins (e.g., albumin) and body habitus. A higher proportion of adipose tissue relative to total body water can be found in most older adults compared to younger adults [5, 7]. Therefore, Vd is increased for lipophilic medications, resulting in a longer half-life and increased potential for side effects. Frail, older patients might have low protein levels due to conditions such as chronic kidney or liver disease or malnutrition. In these frail patients, a higher-than-anticipated medication effect might occur with protein-bound medications [4].

Hepatic Metabolism

The liver is the primary site of metabolism of many dermatologic drugs [8]. There are two primary phases of drug metabolism in the liver, but only Phase I reactions (e.g., hydroxylation, oxidation, alkylation, and reduction) are affected by aging [4, 5]. Drugs are converted by Phase I reactions into less pharmacologically active metabolites that are more readily eliminated. Not all medications metabolized by Phase I reactions are necessarily equally affected by age. This heterogeneity may occur because different medications are extracted by the liver to differing degrees [9]. Cytochrome P450 (CYP), which is estimated to process over three-quarters of medications, is a prototypical phase I reaction [5]. CYP content may be reduced by about one-third in humans 70 years of age compared to younger patients [10]. CYP activity can also be altered by common medications and ingestants, including grapefruit juice, antihypertensives, lipid-lowering medications, and some antibiotics (see Table 1) [8, 11].

Renal Clearance

Renal impairment affects at least 10 % of community-dwelling and 40 % of long-term care facility adults ≥65 years and older [12, 13]. Kidney function declines with normal senescence—a 30 % decrease in glomerular filtration rate (GFR) occurs between the ages of 30–80 years—as well as other factors such as nephrotoxic medications and comorbidity complications (e.g., diabetes, hypertension) [14, 15]. Since over 25 % of all human medications have been estimated to be mostly excreted by the kidneys, the prescribing practitioner should be aware when renal dose adjustments are necessary (see Table 1) [4].

A major challenge is determining whether older adults have clinically significant renal disease. Absolute serum creatinine level and/or blood urea nitrogen (BUN) have conventionally been used by clinicians as surrogate markers of renal function. These markers, however, are inaccurate in older adults [16]. Very old patients, particularly frail patients, tend to have decreased muscle mass and creatinine production [14]. Thus, some older adults might have a deceptively "normal" serum creatinine when in fact there is renal insufficiency. Serum creatinine and blood urea nitrogen (BUN) in isolation should not be used to estimate renal function (LOE IV) [16].

Creatinine clearance has often been calculated using the Cockroft–Gault equation as an estimate of GFR. This method has traditionally been used by the Food and Drug Administration (FDA) for renal-dose adjustment recommendations [17]. However, this equation's accuracy, particularly when used for older patients, was called into question [18]. Furthermore, modern creatinine assays are different from when the Cockroft–Gault equation was developed. As a result, this equation might lead to the overestimation of renal function by up to 40 % [17].

There are several currently used or newer measures of renal function. The estimated GFR (eGFR) using the Modification of Diet in Renal Disease (MDRD) formula is reasonably accurate for most non-acute patients, as long as the patient's weight is not extreme (e.g., amputee,

Table 1 Common dermatologic medications that might require dose adjustment, interact with other common medications, or have other potentially adverse effects in older adult patients

Medication	Renal dose adjustment	Cytochrome P450 metabolism	Pharmacokinetic notes	Example of medication interaction	Potential consequences in older patients
Acyclovir	Y				Delirium, nephrotoxicity
H1-antagonists (particularly first generation antihistamines)		Diphenhydramine is potent CYP2D6 inhibitor [39][f]	Hydroxyzine is very lipophilic and has prolonged half-life in older patients	Counteracts cholinesterase inhibitors (might aggravate dementia or cause delirium)	Constipation, delirium
Azathioprine	Y			Decreases warfarin levels	
Benzodiazepines					Excessive sedation, falls, delirium, fractures
Cephalosporins	Cephalexin			Many cephalosporins increase warfarin levels	
Cetirizine	Y				
Chloroquine	Y				Unknown if older patients, especially with existing macular degeneration or renal insufficiency, are at higher risk than younger healthy adults for ocular toxicity
Cimetidine				Increases warfarin levels	
Ciprofloxacin	Y	CYP1A2 inhibitor[f]		If taken with systemic corticosteroids, increases tendon rupture risk. Increases warfarin levels	Prolonged QTc, delirium, and tendon rupture (especially if taken with systemic corticosteroids)
Colchicine	Y				
Cyclosporine	Y	Metabolized by CYP3A3/3A4[f]		Increases digoxin levels	Nephrotoxicity risk
Dapsone		Metabolized by CYP3A3/3A4[f]			May cause hemolytic anemia, which might not be tolerated in patients with cardiopulmonary disease or baseline anemia[a]

(continued)

Table 1 (continued)

Medication	Renal dose adjustment	Cytochrome P450 metabolism	Pharmacokinetic notes	Example of medication interaction	Potential consequences in older patients
Dicloxacillin				Decreases warfarin levels	
Erythromycin		CYP3A4/3A5 inhibitor[f]		Increases warfarin levels	
Famciclovir	Y			Increases warfarin levels	
Fluconazole	Y	CYP2C9 inhibitor[f]		Increases warfarin levels	
Gabapentin	Y		Taper rather than abruptly stop so as to prevent withdrawal[b]		Recommend initiating at 100 mg QHS with slow titration to prevent ataxia and somnolence.
Griseofulvin		Weak/moderate CYP1A2/2C9/3A4 inducer[f]		Decreases warfarin levels	
Itraconazole		CYP3A4/3A5 inhibitor[f]		Increases digoxin levels	
Ketoconazole		CYP3A4/3A5 inhibitor[f]			
Loratadine			Though a second generation non-sedating antihistamine, it is considered anticholinergic by an American Geriatrics Society expert panel and should be used cautiously [41]		Loratadine probably has less anticholinergic effects compared to cetirizine
Macrolides				Increases warfarin levels (except for azithromycin) Increases digoxin levels	
Methotrexate	Y			Caution with trimethoprim, penicillins, nonsteroidal anti-inflammatory drugs (NSAIDs)[c]	

Metronidazole				Increases warfarin levels	May cause dysgeusia and aggravate anorexia in frail patients
Nafcillin				Decreases warfarin levels	
Opioids			Many are hepatically metabolized		Delirium, falls, sedation, constipation [44]. Use low dose and carefully titrate. Recommend scheduled bowel regimen.
Prednisone		Weak/moderate CYP2C19/3A4 inducer[f]			Hypertension, hyperglycemia, osteoporosis, delirium, psychosis, heart failure exacerbation, dysrhythmias, myopathy. Peptic ulcer risk increased 15-fold with concomitant nonsteroidal anti-inflammatory drug (NSAID) (See Table 3)
Ranitidine	Y				
Rifampin		Potent inducer of many CYPs[f]		Decreases warfarin levels	
Terbinafine	Y	CYP2D6 inhibitor[f]			May cause dysgeusia and aggravate anorexia in frail patients
Tetracycline	Y			Increases digoxin levels	
Tricyclic antidepressants (e.g., amitriptyline, doxepin > 6 mg/day)			Taper rather than abruptly stop so as to prevent withdrawal[d]	Counteracts cholinesterase inhibitors (might aggravate dementia or cause delirium)	Delirium, orthostatic hypotension, constipation

(continued)

Table 1 (continued)

Medication	Renal dose adjustment	Cytochrome P450 metabolism	Pharmacokinetic notes	Example of medication interaction	Potential consequences in older patients
Trimethoprim—sulfamethoxazole	Y	CYP2C9 inhibitor[f]			May cause anemia, which might not be tolerated in patients with cardiopulmonary disease or baseline anemia[c]
Tumor necrosis factor (TNF) inhibitors					Might increase skin cancer risk, contraindicated in patients with severe symptomatic heart failure[c,e]
Valacyclovir	Y				

Adapted from Endo et al. 2013 [8] except where indicated

[a]Figueiredo MS, Pinto BO, Zago MA. Dapsone-induced haemolytic anaemia and agranulocytosis in a patient with normal glucose-6-phosphate-dehydrogenase activity. *Acta haematologica.* 1989;82(3):144–145

[b]Green CB, Stratman EJ. Prevent rather than treat postherpetic neuralgia by prescribing gabapentin earlier in patients with herpes zoster: comment on "incidence of postherpetic neuralgia after combination treatment with gabapentin and valacyclovir in patients with acute herpes zoster". *Arch Dermatol.* Aug 2011;147(8):908

[c]C.F. L, L.L. A, M.P. G, L.L. L. *Lexi-Comp Drug Information Handbook.* 20th ed. Hudson, OH: Lexi-Comp; 2011

[d]Labbate LA. Drugs for the treatment of depression. *Handbook of psychiatric drug therapy.* 6th ed. Philadelphia: Wolters Kluwer Health/Lippincott Williams & Wilkins; 2010:xiv, 304 p

[e]Targownik LE, Bernstein CN. Infectious and malignant complications of TNF inhibitor therapy in IBD. *The American journal of gastroenterology.* Dec 2013;108(12):1835–1842, quiz 1843

[f]Examples of cytochrome (CYP) substrate medications in geriatric patients include CYP2C9 (e.g., carvedilol, celecoxib, glipizide, losartan, irbesartan), CYP2C19 (e.g., omeprazole), CYP2D6 (e.g., carvedilol, donepezil, metoprolol), CYP3A4/CYP3A5 (e.g., amlodipine, atorvastatin, cyclosporine, dapsone, estradiol, simvastatin, sildenafil, verapamil, zolpidem)

obese, frail) (LOE IIB) [15, 19]. Further evidence is needed before CKD-EPI and cystatin C will be feasible, widely accepted alternatives to MDRD for older patients (LOE III) [15, 19]. A 24-h urine creatinine clearance collection, despite practical limitations in accurate collection, can be considered in some patients (e.g., extremely high or low weight or amputees) who are taking medicines with a narrow therapeutic window (e.g., methotrexate) (LOE IV) [17].

Pharmacodynamics of Aging

Aging is generally associated with decreased homeostatic functional reserve [9]. The extent of this decrease, which depends on individual genetic makeup, environmental exposures, and comorbidities, can vary greatly between patients. Very old and frail patients are at particularly high risk for experiencing cardiovascular, urinary, and neuropsychiatric side effects [20]. The so-called geriatric syndromes – symptoms that are commonly but inaccurately attributed to the "normal" aging process (e.g., incontinence, falls, or delirium) – are considered by some experts to be preventable patient safety events that are usually caused by adverse medication reactions [21, 22]. However, if a patient has multiple comorbidities that overlap with potential medication side effects, it can be particularly challenging to determine whether a patient's underlying comorbidity is truly progressing or whether iatrogenesis (medication side effect) has occurred [23]. This section discusses common examples of how geriatric syndromes can be caused by dermatologic medications. Special considerations for anticipating and managing immunosuppressant side effects in older adults are also presented.

Geropharmacology might seem far removed from day-to-day clinical reality, but the aforementioned principles have several important implications for commonly prescribed dermatologic medications. While an exhaustive overview of all dermatologic medications is beyond the scope of this chapter, common examples of pitfalls and a number of prescribing pearls are listed in Tables 1, 2, and 3.

Geriatric Syndromes

Benign prostatic hyperplasia (BPH), which is estimated to affect about 70 % of men by the seventh decade of life, can lead to incontinence and/or occasionally bladder obstruction [24]. Urinary symptoms from BPH can be exacerbated by anticholinergic medications, due to the effect on bladder function [25]. Since urge incontinence has been associated with falls and quality of life, medications with anticholinergic effects (e.g., first-generation antihistamines, tricyclic antidepressants) should be avoided (LOE III) [26].

Delirium, an acute confusional state with an alteration of consciousness and attention, is considered a multifactorial syndrome [27]. Although it has been defined as a reversible condition, delirium has been associated with morbidity and mortality and is preventable in many cases [28]. Medications such as narcotics, benzodiazepines, and anticholinergic agents (e.g., tricyclic antidepressants, first-generation antihistamines) are known to cause delirium in the older population. These medications should be avoided altogether or given at very low doses, if they are necessary, especially in patients who already have baseline cognitive impairment (LOE III) [29].

Falls, another multifactorial syndrome, are associated with morbidity and mortality in about 10 % of cases [30]. In patients with preexisting balance instability or a history of falls, decreasing the total number of medications and eliminating medicines that aggravate postural hypotension or alter cognition (see Table 1) are recommended (LOE II) [29, 30].

Special Pharmacodynamic Considerations with Systemic Immunosuppressive Agents

Healthy aging is associated with immunosenescence, which is the age-related alteration of the innate and adaptive immune system [2, 31]. Therefore, older adults are at higher risk for developing infections. This infection risk is further increased when older adults are prescribed immunosuppressants. Older adults might also be at increased risk for having side effects such as osteoporosis or heart failure due to preexisting comorbidities (e.g., osteopenia, coronary disease) or frailty (see Tables 1, 2, and 3).

Table 2 Summary of recommendations to avoid prescription misadventures, including level of evidence (LOE)

Recommendation	Strategies	Comment	LOE
1. If feasible during visit, reassess for medication or health status changes	Periodically review medications using the "brown bag" method	• Patients might be reluctant to acknowledge CAM use • Specifically ask about CAM and over-the-counter drugs, which patients might not consider to be medicines	IV
	Ask patient if they have experienced any hospitalizations, new or worsened medical problems, or other changes in health-care goals		IV
2. Determine if existing drugs can be discontinued or tapered	If patient is tolerating and benefitting from a "high risk medication" it should not be automatically discontinued per se	• See Table 1 for high risk medications	IV
	If patient has an eczematous eruption, discontinue topical antibiotics, fragrance mixes, vitamin E, lanolin, diphenhydramine, or propylene glycol, which are common culprits		IV
	If patient reports worsening rash or stinging after application, consider switching to a different molecule or propylene glycol-free formulation or referring for skin patch testing		III, IV
	If patient is at risk for falling, try to minimize medications that might contribute	• Tricyclic antidepressants • First-generation antihistamines • Benzodiazepines • Anticonvulsants	II, IV
	If stopping or tapering a medicine, do so at the same rate that it would be up-titrated	• Tricyclic antidepressants and gabapentin can cause withdrawal symptoms	IV
3. If new medicine added, carefully consider necessity and risk	If a feasible non-pharmacologic (or non-systemic) option exists, try this before a prescription and/or systemic agent		IV
	If medicine is "high-risk," avoid or minimize use	• See Table 1	III
	If alternatives have failed or are less appropriate in the prescribing context, a trial of a "high-risk medicine" at a very low dose with careful monitoring might be considered		
	If patient prescribed medium-to-high potency steroid, counsel avoiding intertriginous areas or on a chronic, daily basis	• Commonly prescribed antifungal medications (e.g., Lotrisone) might also contain steroids	IV
	If patient has cardiopulmonary disease or baseline anemia, exercise caution in medications that might cause anemia	• Methotrexate • Dapsone (even with normal glucose-6-phosphate-dehydrogenase • Sulfa antibiotics	IV
	If prescribing an immunosuppressive agent, consider prophylaxis	• See Table 3	IV

(continued)

Table 2 (continued)

Recommendation	Strategies	Comment	LOE
4. Identify potential medication interactions	If new medicine is anticipated to interact with a non-dermatologic medicine, notify the patient and other prescribing provider	• Example includes antibiotics interacting with warfarin and needing to counsel patient and anticoagulation prescriber (See Table 1)	IV
	If unsure of drug interactions, use a drug reference	• Electronic medical record • Software • Textbook • Pharmacist	IV
5. Consider if patient is physically able to take the medication or afford the cost	If patient nonadherent or seems reluctant to try medicine, inquire about financial concerns	• Patient might benefit from cheaper formulary option or prescription assistance program (See Appendix) • Most government prescription programs are excluded from manufacturer discount cards	IV
	If patient has a disability or complex regimen that might interfere with adherence, consider assistive devices or other resources	• Pill cutters • Medication organizers (e.g., pill boxes, prepackaged and preorganized blister packs) with time of day reminders • Arthritis-friendly easy-open containers • Large-print labels • Back lotion applicators	IV
	If patient suspected of aspirating, refer to speech therapy or swallow evaluation or consider parenteral administration	• Prior stroke or other neurologic conditions might increase risk	IV
6. Assess whether patient and caregiver understand treatment plan	If patient seems hard-of-hearing, speak in a slow, low tone facing patient	• Sometimes difficulty understanding might be inferred as cognitive impairment when it is actually sensory impairment (e.g., vision or hearing difficulty)	IV
	If the patient has visual impairment, use large-print instructions and include medication addition, discontinuation, indications, and key instructions	• 12-Point font or larger • High color contrast between lettering and paper • Avoid typing in all capital letters	IV
	If patient needs to ask questions or discuss a side effect, provide patient and care giver contact information		IV
	If patient adherence is in question despite above measures, assess decision-making capacity	• Ask the patient to "teach back" key instructions or changes • Mini-mental status exam is a poor discriminatory of capacity except at extreme scores • Aid to Capacity Evaluation (ACE) is a free tool that has the best validity evidence, but requires training • Referral to a geriatrics memory assessment clinic	III, IV

(continued)

Table 2 (continued)

Recommendation	Strategies	Comment	LOE
7. Consider whether patients with comorbidities might require medication dose adjustment and/or slow titration	If a medicine is cleared through kidneys, make sure renal function recently assessed	• Especially for medications with narrow therapeutic index (e.g., methotrexate) recommend conservative dosing • Educate patient on potential delay to effect • Modification of Diet in Renal Disease (MDRD) is generally reasonable estimate, unless patient is amputee, obese or frail • 24-h-urine creatinine clearance may be considered in patients who have extremely high or low weight or an amputee and taking medicines with a narrow therapeutic window • CKD-EPI and cystatin C equations are newer methods that require further validity evidence and availability before practical, widespread use can be recommended	IIB, III, IV
8. Decide whether care coordination with other providers or strategic follow up is needed	If patient on multiple medications is exhibiting geriatric syndrome, and/or there is concern about their decision-making capacity, consider geriatrics referral	• Interdisciplinary medication management (pharmacist, case manager)	IV
	If drug interaction anticipated, communicate medication changes with primary care provider and/or other specialists	• Primary provider often helpful for mobilizing additional resources, providing insight into patient's psychosocial situation	IV
	If adherence in question or medication needs close monitoring, strategically schedule follow up	• Schedule next appointment (perhaps nurse visit) few weeks after dose adjustment/change • Periodic staff follow up calls or patient reminder letters • Ensure visits of sufficient length to answer questions, have clinical staff assist with patient education	IV

Review and/or renegotiate patient and caregiver goals within the context of comorbidities, life expectancy, and psychosocial context. Refer to text for references

Systemic Corticosteroid Side Effects and Prophylaxis

Systemic steroids have a plethora of side effects, including opportunistic infections, ulcers, hyperglycemia, hypertension, delirium, glaucoma, heart failure, weakness from myopathy, arrhythmias, cataracts, osteopenia, and osteoporosis [32]. Although these side effects are not geriatric syndromes per se, the same principles of cautious prescribing and close monitoring also apply to systemic corticosteroids. Careful patient education

Table 3 Prophylaxis recommendations when prescribing immunosuppressants to older adult patients

Immunosuppressant	Recommendation	Comment	LOE
All immunosuppressants	If "intensive" immunosuppression anticipated, try to administer *live* vaccines (e.g., shingles) at least 4 weeks in advance of immunosuppression, if possible		IV
	If patient given immunosuppressants, consider administering *killed* virus vaccines (e.g., pneumococcal)	• No reason to withhold *killed* virus vaccines from immunosuppressed patients, though seroconversion rates might be lower	IV
	If patient already has chronic immunosuppressing condition or taking two or more immunosuppressants, consider pneumocystis pneumonia prophylaxis	• Trimethoprim-sulfamethoxazole, atovaquone, dapsone, or pentamidine	IV
Systemic glucocorticoids	Coordinate with primary care or other specialists to monitor glucose, blood pressure, ocular pressure	• Especially in patients with known risk factors (e.g., impaired fasting glucose, congestive heart failure)	IV
	Osteoporosis prevention should be considered for patients with other bone risk factors	• The American College of Rheumatology published recommendations for preventing glucocorticoid-induced osteoporosis (see Appendix for risk stratification and recommendations for vitamin D, calcium, bone density monitoring, lifestyle counseling)	IV
	Peptic ulcer disease prophylaxis	• H2-receptor antagonist or proton pump inhibitor (along with limited alcohol intake) should be considered, especially in patients with a history of peptic ulcer, heavy alcohol intake, or anticoagulant use • Withhold aspirin or nonsteroidal anti-inflammatory drug (NSAID) use, if possible	IV
Azathioprine Methotrexate Systemic glucocorticoids	If patient already taking more than prednisone 20 mg daily equivalent dose, methotrexate 0.4 mg/kg/week, or azathioprine 3 mg/kg/day avoid live virus (e.g., zoster) vaccines		IV
	If immunocompetent household member receives zoster vaccine and develops cutaneous lesions, avoid close contact with immunocompromised patients		IV
Rituximab	If patient receives influenza vaccine within 6 months of infusion, vaccine benefit might be low		IV
Azathioprine Cyclosporine Mercaptopurine Tumor necrosis factor (TNF) antagonists	If patient receiving chronic therapy with these agents, consider annual skin cancer screening	• Particularly important to offer skin cancer screening in immunosuppressed patients who also have a personal history of skin cancers/precancers or family history of skin cancers	IV

and coordination of care with the primary care provider or relevant specialists (e.g., cardiologist, ophthalmologist, diabetologist) are recommended prior to and during systemic steroid treatment (LOE IV).

Since hip fracture in older adults is associated with a fivefold increased 3-month mortality risk and morbidity compared to those without fracture, it is important to understand osteoporosis risk and prevention strategies in patients taking corticosteroids [33]. A meta-analysis demonstrated that patients taking a prednisone dose as low as 7.5 mg daily had an increased risk of fracture [34]. The American College of Rheumatology (ACR) published updated guidelines in 2010 (see Appendix for risk tables and algorithm), which provide evidence-based recommendations for monitoring and managing patients who are taking prednisone [35]. They recommend stratifying an individual patient's risk of fracture based on patient characteristics (e.g., alcohol intake, tobacco use, history of fracture, race, gender, height and weight, baseline hip bone density) and anticipated duration and dose of steroid. Based on this calculated risk, the prescribing provider can determine if lifestyle counseling (including vitamin D and calcium doses), prophylaxis with bisphosphonates, and bone density and height monitoring are appropriate (LOE IV).

Recently, there has been controversy over whether corticosteroid monotherapy is associated with an increased risk of peptic ulcers and GI bleeding. Some experts have argued that GI prophylaxis should not be given for glucocorticoid monotherapy, regardless of dose [32]. A systematic review and meta-analysis demonstrated that peptic ulcer risk is indeed increased (odds ratio 1.43, 95% CI 1.22–1.66) for subjects taking corticosteroids compared to placebo [36]. Subgroup analysis suggested that inpatients, but not ambulatory patients, have a statistically significantly increased risk for ulcers. While this study did not make specific recommendations about GI prophylaxis, it acknowledged that most studies included in the analysis did not specify whether subjects took GI prophylaxis and there was no specific subgroup analysis by age. However, the current authors contend that older patients are generally at higher risk for GI bleeding—probably for multi-

ple reasons, including age-associated changes of GI mucosa, prevalence of *H. pylori* carriage, and anticoagulant and nonsteroidal anti-inflammatory drug (NSAID) use [37]. Furthermore, older adults who experience GI bleeding have higher mortality rates than do younger adults. Therefore, it is the current authors' recommendation that GI prophylaxis (H2 receptor antagonist or proton pump inhibitor) should be strongly considered in older adult patients who are taking systemic steroids, particularly if they have a history of GI bleeds, heavy alcohol ingestion, or take anticoagulants, aspirin, or NSAIDs (LOE IV). Aspirin or NSAIDs should be suspended, unless there is a major contraindication to doing so (LOE IV).

Infectious Disease Prophylaxis

Infectious disease prophylaxis is important when prescribing chronic systemic steroids or other immunosuppressants, but preventive measures are particularly important in older adults. During normal aging, there is decreased epidermal barrier function against pathogens and impairment of cell-mediated immunity (immunosenescence), which might predispose patients to many skin conditions and infections [31]. Many older adults also have comorbid cardiopulmonary or renal diseases, which further increase immunosuppression [38–41]. Most of the discussion here centers on systemic steroids, though many principles are generalized to other steroid-sparing agents. The authors focus on the more common and serious viral, fungal, and bacterial infections and discuss strategies to mitigate the risk.

Herpes zoster (shingles) tends to occur with aging due to reactivation of dormant varicella zoster virus that occurs as a consequence of immunosenescence [42]. This condition can cause significant morbidity (e.g., postherpetic neuralgia, herpes zoster ophthalmicus) [43]. The risk of zoster is probably increased in patients taking systemic corticosteroids [44]. Zoster vaccination is recommended as part of health-care maintenance for patients 50 years and older and would ideally occur before the need for systemic immunosuppression. However, one study showed that about one-sixth of eligible patients receive the vaccine [45]. According to the Infectious Disease Society of America (IDSA), this live virus vaccine should not be given to patients taking more than prednisone 20 mg daily, methotrexate 0.4 mg/kg/week, or azathioprine 3 mg/kg/day (LOE IV) [46]. If patients are to be prescribed more intensive immunosuppression, the ACR recommends waiting until at least 4 weeks after zoster immunization, when possible (LOE IV) [42]. Immunocompetent household contacts over 60 years of age may be given the vaccine, but they should avoid close contact with the patient if skin lesions develop (LOE IV) [46].

There is a paucity of data for making influenza vaccination recommendations in patients taking chronic steroids or other immunosuppressants. About half of such studies suggest that patients can mount an immunogenic response [47]. Although the specific risk of influenza from chronic steroid or other immunosuppressant use is poorly characterized, the IDSA recommends that patients receive influenza vaccination (only the inactivated intramuscular type, not live attenuated) on an annual basis (LOE IV) [46]. Patients receiving influenza vaccine within 6 months of rituximab are unlikely to seroconvert and unlikely to be harmed, but the IDSA recommends against administering the vaccine in such cases (LOE IV) [46]. Similarly, pneumococcal vaccination is recommended for chronically immunosuppressed patients, though these patients might have a blunted seroconversion titer (LOE IV) [46].

Pneumocystis jirovecii pneumonia (formerly P. carinii or "PCP", now called PJP) is an opportunistic fungal infection. There are limited data to support PJP prophylaxis in immunocompromised patients without human immunodeficiency virus (HIV). It should be noted that most published recommendations for prophylaxis were based on uncontrolled studies or expert opinion and did not necessarily include patients prescribed immunosuppression for a primary skin condition, and did not specify whether age per se was an independent risk factor for developing PJP. While PJP is known to have potentially adverse outcomes, especially in HIV-negative patients, experts differ in their recommended indications for which patients on chronic immunosuppression should receive prophylaxis [48]. For instance, some recommend that a 16–20 mg daily prednisone dose should warrant PJP prophylaxis (LOE III, IV) [49, 50]. Others suggest that patients should receive prophylaxis if they take 20 mg prednisone daily for over 1 month and have another immunosuppressing comorbidity or medication (LOE III, IV) [51]. Still others contend that chronic steroid patients with certain CD4 or total lymphocyte counts (LOE III), or interstitial lung disease (LOE IV), or chronic anti-TNF therapy alone or in combination with steroids should receive PJP prophylaxis (LOE IV) [52, 53]. The most convincing systematic review and meta-analysis to date by Green et al. suggests that patients with inflammatory and autoimmune dermatologic conditions who take chronic immunosuppressants probably have a PJP risk that does not outweigh potential side effects from prophylaxis [54]. Based on the available literature, the current authors recommend (LOE IV) considering prophylaxis in patients with chronic immunosuppressing condition (e.g., diabetes, cancer, pulmonary disease), or in those taking two or more immunosuppressants (e.g., chronic prednisone bridging to a steroid-sparing immunosuppressant). The preferred prophylaxis regimen is trimethoprim-sulfamethoxazole (LOE IB), although atovaquone (LOE II), dapsone (LOE II) or pentamidine (LOE IV) may be used [50, 51, 54].

Skin Cancer Monitoring with Tumor Necrosis Factor (TNF) Antagonists

Skin cancer risk has been associated with age, skin type, and certain types of immunosuppressant use [55]. Traditionally, the most commonly associated immunosuppressants with skin cancer risk have been azathioprine and cyclosporine based on solid organ transplant patient data [56]. However, data also suggest that anti-TNF agents and chronic prednisone might increase skin cancer risk, although perhaps not as much as the other immunosuppressants [56, 57]. Extrapolating from the above studies, the current authors recommend annual skin checks in patients receiving chronic thiopurine, cyclosporine, or anti-TNF therapy (LOE IV).

Ethical Considerations of Prescribing to Older Adults

Ethical dilemmas are usually thought of as situations that involve grave life or death scenarios. However, there are ethical considerations when one is prescribing to older adults. The four tenets of medical ethics are autonomy, beneficence, non-maleficence, and justice [58]. Autonomy is defined as the right of rational individuals to make an independent and informed decision about their care. Beneficence is defined as acting in the best interest of the patient. Non-maleficence is not inflicting harm, such as avoiding adverse drug events (ADEs). Justice is defined as the fair treatment of individuals and groups and corresponds to the prescriber being a responsible steward of limited health-care resources. These four tenets are used as a framework to discuss dermatology medication management issues that might be encountered when prescribing to older adults.

To what extent should the elderly and/or their caregivers be allowed to manage their medications, especially when age-related issues such as cognitive impairment may be present? Not all patients are equally autonomous, since this is contingent upon decision-making capacity. Local laws vary as to the definition of "capacity to consent." [59, 60] Generally, legal definitions include the patient's "ability to understand the relevant information about proposed [treatments], appreciate their situation, use reason to make a decision, and communicate their choice" [59, 60]. Incapacity is uncommon among healthy, community-dwelling older adults but is probably underrecognized in the general geriatric population [60]. In one pooled analysis study, the diagnosis of incapacity was missed by over half of health-care providers [60]. Possible reasons to explain this underrecognition of incapacity might include health providers giving patients the benefit of the doubt, lacking training to assess capacity, or erroneously interpreting patient acquiescence (i.e., agreeing to treatment does not mean the patient understood the implications of their decision).

The prescriber must carefully balance clinical judgment and intended beneficence with patient autonomy. The potential dilemma of medical paternalism is aptly summarized by Fontanella et al. "The issue that professionals face, especially in the geriatric medical context, is how to ethically determine what represents merely adverse personal choice and what is neglect founded in incapacity?" [61]. The dermatology provider often provides longitudinal care for older adult patients and might gain a sense of familiarity with patient and caregiver goals. However, the provider must exercise caution against complacently assuming authority of a patient's decisions through unintentional paternalism. A later section discusses the dynamic nature of patient goals and prescribing contexts.

A patient's social support system might be helpful in achieving treatment adherence and health-care access. For instance, older adults might rely on family or friends to counsel them about health-care decisions, to provide transportation, to overcome language or cultural barriers, or to pay for health-care services and medications [62]. However, dilemmas may arise when the patient's treatment goals differ from that of the people who provide the social support network. That is, if the patient is overly deferential to their social support network for fear of retribution or offending their family and friends, the patient's autonomy might be decreased as a result.

Is it ethical to ration limited health-care resources by withholding certain treatments from patients based on age? Another example of medical paternalism is ageism, which is a perceived futility of treatment for adults beyond a certain age. Often, ageism stems from the notion that age is a surrogate of life expectancy, which in turn can be inferred to determine whether limited health-care resources should be reserved instead for patients with longer life expectancy [62, 63]. Providers might have justifiable prescribing standards that differ based on the patient's context, which might include age. As an extreme example, aggressive cutaneous chemopreventive measures may not be wanted or needed by frail older patients with multiple comorbidities and end-of-life care goals.

However, many older adult dermatology patients are often not such outliers, and it is important to avoid ageist prescribing approaches. An individual patient's life span and quality of life, both of which may be improved by prescriptions, are not necessarily reflected by actuarial statistics that provide information about population-based life expectancy [64]. Thus, the current authors recommend that prescription decisions are made after considering the individual patient's context (i.e., not only chronologic age) (LOE IV). The authors also recommend negotiating realistic treatment goals with the patient that are within the confines of limited health-care resources. Potential risks and benefits of each intervention should be considered (LOE IV).

As a corollary to this point, older patients, particularly the frail, have been excluded or underrepresented in most clinical trials [65]. Older patients might be at risk for medication interactions or adverse effects due to comorbidities or functional limitations [62, 63]. However, without adequate safety and dosing data, it can be difficult to assess the cost-effectiveness or potential harms in treating older patients [62, 63]. The tenets of justice, beneficence, and non-maleficence are in conflict due to this evidence gap.

In summary, geriatric ethical dilemmas may arise anywhere from pharmaceutical research and development exclusion criteria all the way to the prescriber's discussion and selection of medications. The above examples highlight the delicacy that is required in balancing autonomy, beneficence, non-maleficence, and justice as well as the complex interplay that exists among the individual patient, caregivers, and society. Later sections further illustrate these ethical issues in geriatric prescribing.

Medication Errors in Older Adult Patients

A significant economic burden and potentially negative patient outcomes can result from medication management errors. This topic is particularly relevant to the geriatric population, which consumes about 42 % of total drug expenditures and is at higher risk for developing ADEs [3, 66]. Hospitalization rates, costs, and length of stay are all increased by ADEs [67]. The total cost of preventable ADEs has been estimated at more than $100 billion per year, or around 10 % of annual American health-care expenditures [68]. While there are several published definitions and categories of medication errors, the authors have adapted a framework by Gupta et al. [69]. Medication errors, or unintended consequences of prescription medications, include inappropriate use, overuse, underprescribing, and medication nonadherence. Previously discussed geropharmacological and ethical principles are applied to the description of these four types of medication errors.

Inappropriate Use

A prescription is deemed inappropriate if the potential risk of utilizing that drug or intervention supersedes the potential for benefit [70]. Geriatricians consider certain medications to be potentially inappropriate and "high risk" for causing adverse reactions in older patients. The Beers criteria is one common reference that lists medications to avoid or use cautiously in older patients (LOE IV). One common example is anticholinergic medications (e.g., amitriptyline, diphenhydramine, and hydroxyzine). Compared to other patient populations, older adults using anticholinergics are at increased risk for mortality, cognitive impairment, acute glaucoma, and tachycardia [71].

Unfortunately, "high risk" prescribing is not uncommon, and the consequences are numerous. One review found that the median rate of inappropriate medication prescriptions for elderly persons in the primary care setting was 20.5 %, with diphenhydramine and amitriptyline being the most common inappropriately prescribed medications [72]. In another study, annual adjusted medical and total health-care costs for older patients who were prescribed "high risk" medications were significantly higher than for controls [73].

Some forms of inappropriate prescribing might seem innocuous but still have consequences. For instance, dermatophytosis (tinea) is often treated with topical nystatin, which is effective against many species of Candida (yeast) but not against dermatophyte infections [74]. Though unlikely to violate non-maleficence, inappropriate prescribing diminishes the benefit that the patient receives and unjustly wastes health-care resources.

Overuse

Several definitions of overuse or polypharmacy (PP) have been described in the literature, but the authors adapt the definition described by Gupta et al.: "The concomitant use of multiple drugs or the administration of more medications than clinically indicated" [75, 76]. Although an increased number of total medications are associated with more adverse events, an arbitrary cutoff is not recommended by the current authors for two main reasons: taking multiple medications may benefit some patients with multiple comorbidities, and no specific cut off has been validated in the literature [76–78].

PP in dermatology is not uncommon. One study of dermatology patients showed that PP (defined as simultaneous use of ≥ 4 medications) nearly tripled from 5.6 % in 1995 to 18.5 % in 2009. Patients ≥ 65 years were amongst the highest proportion of patients with PP [75]. Several causes of unintentional PP might coexist. For example, the patient might be taking duplicate medications due to confusion between generic and trade drug names. Another instance is when patients mistakenly continue taking medications that were changed by a provider, either due to miscommunication between provider and patient or due to medication reconciliation errors during transitions of care between different health-care providers and settings [8]. PP can become a vicious cycle of iatrogenesis that can develop over time. For example, prescription cascades might occur when one medication is causing an ADE that is misinterpreted as a medical condition and is then treated with more medication [79, 80]. Another variant of PP is when medications from the same class are inadvertently used together to treat the same condition (e.g., hydroxyzine and cetirizine prescribed together for itch, two similar class steroids to treat one anatomic area) [8, 76].

PP can negatively affect older patients in several ways. Medication non-adherence (due to confusion over which medications to take and when) is one of the possible consequences of PP. Additionally, the potential for drug–drug interactions increases due to PP. For instance, potential drug–drug interactions were found in one study to be frequent in hospitalized dermatology patients [81].

Providers should be cognizant of the causes and consequences of PP. However, it is also important to not take an extreme stance and omit potentially beneficial medications. The underprescription of medications is becoming increasingly prevalent, and in some studies has been found to actually be more common than medication overuse [82].

Underprescription

Underprescription has been defined as the omission of drug therapy when use of the medication is indicated for the prevention or treatment of a medical condition [82]. Studies suggest that over half of hospitalized patients, 13 % of nursing home patients, and 22 % of community-dwelling older adults might not be receiving appropriate prescriptions for their medical conditions [82]. Ironically, one study showed that the probability of underprescription increases as the total number of drugs increases [83]. In other words, it is possible that patients take too many dangerous or unnecessary medications but not enough medications that might provide a justifiable benefit.

While some frail patients with multiple comorbidities and medications might benefit from a minimalist prescribing approach, the provider must also mindfully avoid an ageist approach. Other causes of underprescription include fear of perturbing multiple co-morbidities, causing ADEs, economic issues, and a lack of clinical trial data regarding medication use in the elderly population [84]. Although underprescription in other specialties is associated with reduced quality of life and with increased morbidity and mortality in older patients, more studies on how underprescription impacts geriatric dermatology patients are needed [85].

Medication Non-adherence

Medication non-adherence occurs when patients do not take medications in the way that they are prescribed [86]. This phenomenon is not uncommon in older adults. One study showed that agreement between individuals' pharmacy records and self-reported medications tended to be poorer in older than in younger subjects [87]. Unfortunately, patients are not necessarily reliable reporters of non-adherence. One study found that 6 % of dermatology patients self-reported non-adherence, although almost half of prescriptions were unfilled at 2 weeks [88].

Nonadherence is a major problem that can lead to iatrogenesis and increased health-care cost in the elderly population. Up to 21 % of ADEs in older adults in the ambulatory setting were associated with non-adherence in one study [89]. Nonadherence results in drug wastage, which is estimated at more than US$1 billion [90, 91]. Furthermore, patients who "fail" first line therapies might be prescribed more potent and more costly treatments (e.g., topical steroid non-adherence being misinterpreted as refractory disease might result in prescribing systemic therapy).

Several factors are associated with non-adherence. Older patients who take ≥3 medications, especially if each medicine is supposed to be taken on a different scheduling regimen, are at risk for taking incorrect doses of their medications [92]. Physical consequences of aging may also contribute to non-adherence. For instance, patients >65 years old with vision impairment are more likely to have difficulty managing their medications [93]. Arthritis might make it difficult to open bottles, split pills, or apply topical medications to some anatomic sites (see Table 2 for other examples and strategies to overcome these physical disabilities) [6, 8].

Miscommunication between health-care providers and their older patients may also contribute to non-adherence. To illustrate, a sample of community-dwelling Medicare beneficiaries aged 65 and older showed that almost one-third had not spoken with their physician about their medications over the past year [94]. Several studies showed that many older patients failed to understand the purpose of their medications. This lack of understanding is associated with poorer adherence [95]. In particular, frail elderly patients may not feel well-informed or comfortable regarding their medication regimens [96].

Complementary and Alternative Medicine (CAM) Among Older Adult Patients

The terms "complementary" and "alternative" are often used interchangeably to describe non-mainstream health-care approaches. These terms, however, do not mean the same thing. "Complementary" refers to the use of a non-mainstream approach together with conventional medicine [97]. "Alternative" refers to using a non-mainstream approach instead of conventional medicine [97]. CAM generally falls into the category of natural products (e.g., herbs, vitamins, minerals, probiotics) and mind and body practices (where procedures or techniques are administered or taught) [97]. This section focuses on ingested and topical natural products, because these are the most likely to be used to self-treat dermatologic conditions and to cause dermatologic side effects.

CAM use among older Americans is steadily increasing despite limited evidence regarding the safety and efficacy of CAM [98]. One study showed that 14 % of women ≥65 years old took herbs/supplements in 1998 [99]. By 2001, 26.1 % of women ≥65 years reported using supplements. Similarly, supplement use in men ≥65 years old doubled between 2000 and 2001 with 22.7 % of older men using CAM by 2002 [100]. In 2008, a study of adults aged 57–85 years showed that

49 % had used a dietary supplement [101]. The majority of CAM users in dermatology are insured white females who are 50–79 years of age. Of note, adults reporting skin disease are more likely to use CAM (an analysis of the 2007 National Health Interview Survey showed that 84.5 % of patients who reported skin problems in the past year used CAM) than those who do not report skin disease [102].

Several reasons for CAM's popularity have been proposed. Some patients might wish to use CAM as a way to participate in their treatment, control their health and aging process, or resist the "biomedicalization" of aging [103]. Others might have certain causal beliefs about their illness or desire a holistic, natural, or spiritual approach to their health care.

Although many older patients use CAM, they often do not disclose CAM usage to their healthcare providers. One study showed that 46.7 % of older adults in Minnesota did not disclose their CAM usage to their physicians for reasons such as "not being asked" (38.5 %) "didn't think about it" (22 %), and "didn't think it was important to my care" (22 %) [104]. Another study suggested that patients might fear negative views of their CAM usage or feel the need to protect cultural knowledge [105]. These studies indicate that good provider-patient communication is an important part of discussing CAM usage. This theory is supported by another study by Faith et al. which showed that CAM users who had established, positive relationships with their care providers were more likely to disclose CAM use [106]. Additional research is needed regarding how to best inquire about CAM while maintaining therapeutic rapport. The current authors recommend fostering an open, non-judgmental line of questioning (LOE IV) [104, 106, 107]. For example, the prescriber might say: "Many of my patients use herbals, home remedies, or alternative medicines. It's important for me to understand if you are using any of these to provide you with the best care…" The Appendix contains several CAM resources, including patient discussion strategies and how to respond to patients who shun allopathic treatments in favor of CAM.

Patients are often unaware of potential side effects from CAM usage [108–110]. A survey of CAM usage in patients with rosacea and psoriasis revealed that none of the patients were aware of potential CAM side-effects or of the active ingredients. Although touted as natural and safe, CAM has been reported to cause Stevens-Johnson syndrome, arsenic toxicity, allergic dermatologic reactions, photosensitization, Sweet's syndrome, pellagra dermatitis, mercury poisoning, and hypersensitivity reactions [98, 110–112].

CAM interaction with prescription medications is another potential source of harm. A retrospective review of adults aged 60–99 years old demonstrated that potential interactions between supplements and medications were noted for 10/22 of the surveyed supplements [113]. One study showed that licorice can lead to the potentiation of oral and topical corticosteroids, that the Chinese herbal product xaio chai hu tang can lead to decreased blood concentrations of prednisolone, that St. John's Wort can lead to decreased bioavailability of cyclosporine, and that anthranoid-containing plants (including senna and cascara) and soluble fibers (including guar gum and psyllium) can decrease the absorption of drugs [114].

Some natural products are adulterated with corticosteroids [108, 112]. For instance, one analysis found that 8/11 Chinese herbal creams used for the treatment of dermatological conditions contained dexamethasone, while another study found that 38 % of 120 samples of CAM in India were adulterated with steroids [115, 116]. The clinician should recognize steroid-induced side effects from CAM natural products, since patients might not realize they are using a steroid-adulterated product.

In summary, CAM usage in elderly dermatologic patients is common despite the limited data that exist about its safety and efficacy. In some cases, CAM products might interact with prescription medications or contain potentially dangerous additives that can cause a broad range of toxicities or dermatologic conditions. Patients are often unaware of the potential harm that can result from using CAM. Additionally, patients may not disclose their CAM usage to health-care providers.

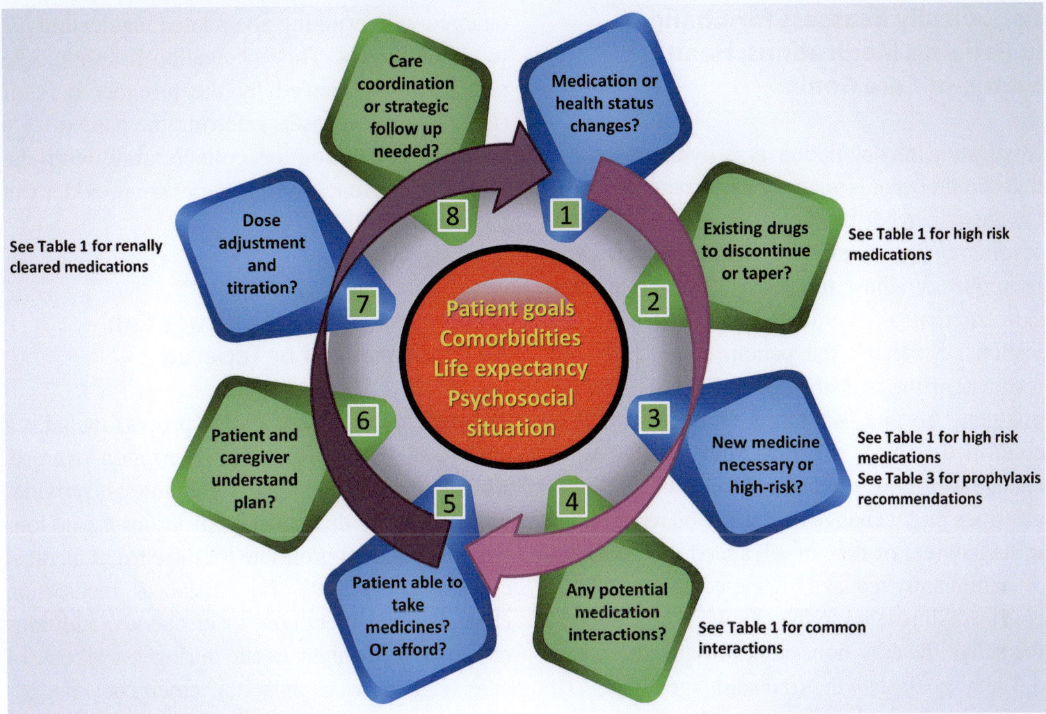

Fig. 1 Prescribing medicines to older dermatology patients is a continuous process that should be centered on patient goals (see also Table 2). (1) Periodically reassess the medication list and monitor for health status changes that might impact treatment goals. (2) Discontinue or taper existing medications if an iatrogenic reaction is suspected or medication no longer indicated. (3) Carefully weigh risk versus benefit of new medicines, especially if it is "high risk." If starting an immunosuppressant, consider prophylaxis. (4) Check for medical interactions, including complementary or alternative medicines and over-the-counter medicines. (5) Ensure the patient is physically able to take the medications and inquire about potential financial concerns. (6) Assess whether the patient and the caregiver understand the treatment plan through clear communication. Decision-making capacity might need to be assessed. (7) Consider whether renal or other dose adjustments are necessary. Start at a low dose and slowly titrate. (8) Decide whether care coordination with other providers is needed. Strategically scheduled follow up visits might improve adherence. Adapted from Garfinkel et al. 2007, Steinman et al. 2010, Lesselroth & Henkel 2012 and Endo et al. 2013

Prescribing Heuristics: The Geriatric Dermatology Prescription Cycle

There are many published tools and guidelines that discuss proposed quality measures of prescribing appropriateness and algorithms for avoiding medication errors. However, several focus on non-dermatology medications or on inpatient settings [71]. The current authors have synthesized recommendations, which are based on the available published evidence, to guide clinicians in prescribing dermatologic medications for older adult patients using best practices (See Fig. 1, Tables 1, 2, and 3). Central to these recommendations is a patient-centered approach that considers the "prescribing context" (i.e., patient and caregiver goals, life expectancy, psychosocial context, and comorbidities). This approach is similar to concepts that have been described by Spinewine et al. [117]. The current authors propose an iterative approach to the prescribing process to reflect the dynamic nature of older patients' health status and the multitude of other prescribing health-care providers who are likely to be involved in older patients' care.

Periodically Reassess for Changes in Patient's Medications, Health Status, or Care Goals

Medication reconciliation is a dynamic process that should occur – not only when new medicines are prescribed but also as an ongoing process – for several reasons. First, other health-care providers prescribe or adjust medicines that might cause skin eruptions or interact with dermatologic medications. Similarly, the patient might also self-medicate using over-the-counter (OTC) or CAM products. Second, patient adherence should be confirmed. Third, the prescribing context can change over time. Patient and caregiver goals and priorities might change or need to be renegotiated in the context of new or advanced comorbidities or significantly reduced life expectancy (LOE IV) [117]. As illustrated in the chapter's introduction, the active, healthy nonagenarian will likely have different goals than the frail septuagenarian.

The current authors have anecdotally observed that solely relying on the "current" electronic medical record medication list might not always be accurate, because patients might receive care from multiple health-care systems. Therefore, to meet the above needs of medication reconciliation, the current authors recommend the "brown bag" method—having patients periodically bring all their OTC, prescription, and CAM products in a bag to be reviewed by the provider or staff (LOE IV) [87]. The current authors recommend that patients should be asked about herbal remedies and OTCs, which patients might consider as benign but could interact with other medicines (LOE IV).

Time constraints in a busy clinic might limit the frequency of such comprehensive reviews and should be customized to the individual patient's situation (LOE IV) [118]. When patients are poor historians or receive prescriptions from multiple pharmacies and adherence is in question, the current authors recommend contacting pharmacists to investigate which medications have been picked up recently (LOE IV). If the provider is unable to contact the pharmacist, clinical staff, medical students or residents can be helpful delegates. The patient or caregiver can be charged with bringing an updated medication list to appointments. This medication list should be periodically reviewed by the provider or staff (LOE). In some cases, referring the patient for a geriatric evaluation or collaborating with the patient's pharmacist or primary care provider can be helpful (LOE IV) [118].

Determine If Existing Drugs Can Be Discontinued or Tapered

The medication reconciliation process includes a critical step in preventing prescription overuse, whenever possible. The dermatology provider might discover that some medications are no longer relevant or appropriate for the current medical context [117, 119]. For instance, medication changes (i.e., intentional or erroneous, additions or omissions) might occur during transitions of care (e.g., between hospital, emergency department, community, nursing home) [120]. New or worsening comorbidities might develop. As a result, the medication dose may need to be changed or discontinued altogether.

When it comes to prescribing to older dermatology patients, less *might* be more [118]. As discussed in the pharmacodynamics and medication errors sections, the risks of polypharmacy should be weighed against the potential for underprescribing. For example, if a patient's care goal is currently being met with the use of a "high-risk medicine" that is not causing any side effects, the medicine should not be discontinued per se (LOE IV). However, it would not be unreasonable to try to titrate the medication to a lower dose (LOE IV) [118]. Common dermatologic medications that might increase the risk for adverse events in older patients are listed in Table 1.

Unfortunately, there are no evidence-based guidelines for how to stop medicines that are irrelevant or causing iatrogenesis. One heuristic is to taper the medicine at about the same rate it would have been up-titrated (LOE IV) [118, 121]. In particular, it is important to counsel patients that abruptly discontinuing tricyclic antidepressants or gabapentin should be avoided to prevent withdrawal (LOE IV) [122, 123].

If a life-threatening or severe adverse reaction is occurring, stopping many or all medications at once can be considered (LOE IV) [118].

Sometimes patients are the unwitting source of iatrogenesis. Patients frequently self-treat with CAM or OTC medications (LOE IV). Many older patients have xerosis or statis dermatitis, which are associated with an increased risk of developing contact dermatitis [124]. In the current authors' experience many patients cause or exacerbate contact dermatitis by using topical medicaments. Common examples include topical antibiotics (e.g., neomycin) and products containing fragrance mixes, vitamin E, lanolin, and diphenhydramine [124, 125]. Thus, the authors generally recommend that patients avoid such products (LOE IV). Patch testing can be helpful in elucidating potential culprit allergens, which on occasion can include an allergy to a topical steroid medication (LOE III) [126]. Sometimes the delivery vehicle instead of the active drug is the cause of contact dermatitis. For example, propylene glycol is found in many prescription and non-prescription agents and can cause contact dermatitis [127]. Empirically switching to a formulation that does not contain propylene glycol can be both diagnostic and therapeutic (LOE IV) [128].

Balance the Risk Versus Benefit of Adding or Adjusting Medications

The prescriber must exercise clinical judgment in deciding whether potentially adding or increasing the dose of a medication will have benefits that outweigh side effects in the prescribing context. Sometimes a reasonable non-pharmacologic treatment option exists. For instance, could the patient's post-procedural pain be treated with an ice pack or low-dose acetaminophen instead of a narcotic (which can cause delirium, constipation, urinary symptoms) or NSAIDs (which can aggravate hypertension or chronic kidney disease) [8, 129]?

If a prescription medication is necessary, consider whether the potential time to expected benefit of the medicine's effect is realistic with respect to the patient's life expectancy [64]. Although one must avoid ageism, it is impossible to judge exactly how long a patient might live. For example, can a prescriber justify prescribing topical 5-fluorouracil as a primary prevention for squamous cell carcinoma in a nonagenarian to meaningfully affect mortality and quality of life?

The practitioner must also consider whether the proposed new medication is "high risk" for causing geriatric syndromes or other major side effects (Tables 1 and 3). Many expert panels recommend generally avoiding these drugs (LOE IV) [29]. As previously mentioned, this recommendation must be balanced against preventing underprescription. It is the current authors' opinion that the clinician might identify extenuating circumstances where a trial of a "high-risk medicine" at a very low dose with careful monitoring might be appropriate in extenuating circumstances, if alternatives have failed or are less appropriate in the prescribing context (LOE IV).

Medium to strong potency steroids deserve special mention for iatrogenesis. On several occasions, the authors have encountered patients with steroid-induced atrophy from chronic, daily application of medium (e.g., triamcinolone) to high (e.g., clobetasol, betamethasone diproprionate, fluocinonide) potency steroids. When topical steroids are applied to intertriginous regions (e.g., under the breasts, groin, axillae, buttocks), atrophy can quickly occur because these areas are thin and occluded [130]. One commonly prescribed combination antifungal and high potency steroid—betamethasone diproprionate/clotrimazole, trade name Lotrisone—is noteworthy. The authors have observed patients referred to dermatology who developed ulcers after inappropriately self-medicating intertriginous areas for presumed fungal infections without realizing that the medication contained a potent steroid. While intermittent topical steroids play an important role in many inflammatory skin conditions, the authors recommend avoiding medium to high potency steroids, including combination antifungal medicines that contain such steroids, in intertriginous areas or on a chronic, daily basis (LOE IV) [131]. The authors also recommend that patients be counseled about the appropriate use of topical steroids (i.e., not applying steroids daily as a "moisturizer" or self-treating other rashes), particularly medium to high potency steroids. In addition to preventing atrophy and ulcers, such patient education might help prevent steroid tachyphylaxis (i.e., diminishing effect due to chronic use beyond just a month or so) (LOE IV).

Immunosuppressants are sometimes necessary to manage severe inflammatory or autoimmune conditions such as bullous pemphigoid. In such cases, a prescription cascade of prophylaxis might be appropriate to offset potential medication side effects, though this must be weighed against potential harms from PP (Table 3) (LOE IV).

Recognize Common Medication Interactions

Several common dermatologic medications used by geriatric patients interact with other prescription medications that might not be managed by the dermatology practitioner (Table 1). For instance, many antibiotics can interact with warfarin [8]. The authors recommend that the prescriber notify the patient and provider managing anticoagulation to determine whether dose adjustment or more frequent monitoring is required (LOE IV). Another common example is that several antifungals can interact with medications that are metabolized via the CYP pathways, thus the authors recommend using a reference (e.g., software, medication book, pharmacist) to verify whether dose adjustments are required (LOE IV) [8]. Several electronic resources are available to check for medication interactions, but common examples are listed in Table 1. The CAM section describes other potential interactions.

Physical Ability to Take Medications and to Afford the Cost

Comorbidities can act as barriers to taking medicines. One common example is hand osteoarthritis, which affects 80 % of older adults and creates physical limitations for adherence (e.g., opening medication packaging, splitting or handling small pills, or self-injecting) [14, 132–134].

Degenerative shoulder or back problems can lead to difficulty in reaching the lower extremities, back, or scalp [8]. Some older adults (e.g., those who suffered a stroke) might be at risk for aspirating. In such cases, the current authors recommend a referral for a swallow study or speech therapy evaluation to find safe ways of taking oral medications (LOE IV) [8]. In some cases, the current authors recommend that parenteral or transdermal routes of administration might be necessary (LOE IV).

For many older patients who might live on a fixed income, prescription costs are a major barrier to adherence. Inability to receive care creates an ethical dilemma of justice. One study estimated that 20 % of patients aged ≥65 years could not afford their medications [134]. While co-pay discount cards seem like a logical solution, these programs often exclude patients who have government sponsored prescription insurance such as Medicaid, TRICARE, or Medicare [8]. Some pharmacies offer low-cost prescription assistance for certain medicines. It can be uncomfortable for patient and prescriber to discuss financial hardships, but the current authors recommend tactfully eliciting patients' concerns about prescription medicines, particularly if anticipated out-of-pocket costs are high (LOE IV).

Patient and Caregiver Understanding of Treatment Plan

It might be assumed that verbal or written explanations lead to patient and caregiver understanding, which in turn would improve adherence. However, several potential communication barriers are outlined in Table 2 along with how these barriers can be overcome. While some might argue that these communication strategies might be too time-consuming, a study has shown that these strategies do not significantly prolong office visits [135]. Furthermore, the potential benefit of avoiding medication errors and achieving intended therapeutic goals justifies using these strategies (LOE IV). Although a Cochrane review did not find that any *single* intervention was effective across all patient populations and contexts to improve adherence, it is plausible that a combination of strategies might be beneficial and theoretically improve informed decision-making (LOE IV) [136]. In a busy clinical setting, many of the following strategies may be potentially delegated to nursing staff.

One particular aspect of patient and care giver understanding is the assessment of decision-making capacity. There are several challenges in assessing capacity. A major challenge is the contextual nature of capacity. Some patients might have limited capacity for low-risk decisions, but not high-stakes circumstances. Additional layers of potential misunderstanding can be created by cultural or language barriers in older patients, such as differently perceived values of health care or level of engagement with the dermatology provider. Capacity is also dynamically altered by temporary factors (e.g., acute illness, delirium) as well as chronic conditions, such as dementia. Thus, capacity for a given patient cannot be extrapolated to every situation that the patient may encounter.

Several tools have been described in the literature. All of these tools, however require some degree of training and none of them have been universally adopted. The commonly used Mini-Mental State Examination (MMSE) is a poor surrogate for assessing capacity except at extremely high or low scores (which are generally obvious to clinicians) (LOE III) [60]. According to one review, the Aid to Capacity Evaluation (ACE), which is also free, is recommended as the best available tool with the most validity evidence (LOE III) [60]. If the practitioner is unable to assess capacity, the authors recommend that the provider refer the patient to a memory or geriatrics clinic (LOE IV).

Dose Adjustment and Titration

The common adage from geriatrics "start low and go slow" is based on the pharmacokinetic principles discussed earlier. Unfortunately, there is often a lack of scientific evidence to guide the appropriate starting dose, target dose, and rate of titration in older adults. Therefore, one must use clinical judgment (LOE IV). Except for life-threatening or urgent conditions, it is generally safest to prescribe at a lower than usual dose (i.e., compared to young, healthy patients), especially with medications such as methotrexate that have narrow therapeutic windows for toxicity (LOE IV) [137]. In addition to counseling patients about potential side effects and providing rationale for a conservative dosing approach, the current authors also recommend explicitly telling patients up front to be patient during the titration process. Setting expectations of care can help maintain therapeutic rapport during the medication adjustments (LOE IV).

As mentioned in the pharmacokinetics section, chronic kidney disease is not uncommon in older adults. Because many medications are renally cleared, it is important to always remember that a "normal" serum creatinine might not reflect normal renal clearance (LOE III). This is especially true in medicines with narrow therapeutic windows. Other comorbid conditions such as chronic anemia, cardiopulmonary disease, and memory impairment might also affect which medicines might be particularly problematic for certain patients (LOE IV).

Coordinate Care and Schedule Strategic Follow Up

Many older adult patients see multiple ambulatory care providers. Even if the prescription rationale is thoughtfully planned and patient-provider communication is superb, medication errors can still occur after the patient leaves the dermatology encounter. In addition to patient factors (e.g., forgetting to take medicines, discontinuing due to side effects), systems-based factors are also potential sources of medication errors. Prescription adjustments made by the dermatology provider might impact other providers (and vice versa), thus an interprofessional, team-based approach is often necessary. The current authors recommend that the primary care provider, case manager or medical director be notified of any medication changes (LOE IV). These providers can be helpful in monitoring medications (e.g., if an antibiotic might interact with warfarin, the primary provider can facilitate more frequent monitoring or dose adjustment), providing key insight into the patient context (e.g., treatment goals, psychosocial situation), and mobilizing additional resources (e.g., home health, interdisciplinary medication management with a pharmacist, formal geriatrics assessment) [138].

Carefully planned office visits are another helpful but potentially overlooked method of maximizing adherence and monitoring in select cases. The current authors recommend that providers reserve longer visit slots or end-of-clinic appointments for patients who are anticipated to have care coordination challenges (e.g., chronic ulcer patients who might need care from a surgeon and wound care clinic, patients who are very hard of hearing) (LOE IV). Strategically timing the interval between office visits can also influence medication adherence. "White coat compliance" describes the increased medication adherence rate that occurs right before follow up appointments [139, 140]. The practitioner might schedule a follow-up visit or call (perhaps in coordination with the primary care provider or home health nurse) as quickly as a week or two after seeing the patient. This action might increase the likelihood that the patient is taking the medication, which in turn might increase the likelihood of achieving the desired therapeutic effect. The provider can also proactively troubleshoot concerns and reinforce the therapeutic alliance with the patient (LOE IV). Of course, practical resource limitations (e.g., staff and provider availability, patient costs) should be considered. These measures might not be routinely feasible in daily practice. However, it is possible with technological advancement (telehealth visits, smartphone applications, and other automated reminder systems) that an effective, individualized "coaching system" might one day become possible.

Summary Points

Aging is a heterogeneous process that is associated with both pharmacokinetic and pharmacodynamic changes. The potential consequences of these age-related changes and how they impact prescribing decisions were reviewed.

Older adult patients (particularly frail patients) often have decreased renal clearance. There are several methods of estimating renal clearance, but relying on absolute serum creatinine alone can be misleading and lead to an overestimation of renal function. Although the Modification of Diet in Renal Disease (MDRD) equation is reliable in most cases, important limitations of MDRD were discussed.

Geriatric patients often have decreased homeostatic physiologic reserve and are therefore at increased risk for adverse drug events.

Geriatric syndromes (e.g., urinary symptoms, delirium, and falls) should not be overlooked, since they can be potentially indicative of iatrogenesis. Medications such as tricyclic antidepressants, first generation antihistamines, and narcotics can all contribute to geriatric syndromes.

Ethical issues related to prescribing, medication research, and assessing patient decision-making capacity were discussed.

Medication errors can be categorized as inappropriate use, overuse, underprescription, and non-adherence. These errors are often multifactorial. The sequelae of these errors include financial burden as well as increased morbidity and mortality for individual patients and for society.

Complementary and alternative medicine (CAM) is commonly used among older dermatology patients for various conditions, including the treatment of dermatologic problems. However, many patients do not readily disclose CAM usage to their health-care providers. Potential prescription medication interactions with CAM and adverse dermatologic manifestations resulting from CAM usage were highlighted.

Prescribing medications should be viewed as a cyclical, dynamic, context-based process that involves the patient, caregivers, and other health-care providers. An evidence-based, best practices prescribing approach was presented. Pertinent examples of dermatologic medications that should be avoided, dosed differently, or prescribed cautiously with close monitoring were also listed. Recommendations for infection, osteoporosis, and peptic ulcer disease prophylaxis were given.

The main geropharmacology research gap is the lack of medication safety, efficacy, and cost-effectiveness data for older adult patients (particularly frail older individuals who are often excluded or underrepresented in clinical trials).

Appendix: Additional Resources

Complementary and Alternative Medicine (CAM)

1. American Association of Clinical Endocrinologists Medical Guidelines for the Clinical Use of Dietary Supplements and Nutraceuticals

    Mechanick JI, Brett EM, Chausmer AB, Dickey RA, Wallach S. American Association of Clinical Endocrinologists Medical Guidelines for the Clinical Use of Dietary Supplements and Nutraceuticals. Endocrine Practice 2003; 9(5): 417–70.

    Authors' Comment: Dietary supplements and nutraceuticals (lists of common supplements and potential interactions are also provided) are defined and discussed in this report. Additionally, strategies and resources that providers can utilize to learn about and discuss dietary supplements and nutraceuticals are provided. Table 8 in this reference lists patient communication strategies for discussing CAM with patients who might be reluctant or belligerent about the topic. Available as free download at https://www.aace.com/files/nutraceuticals-2003.pdf

2. Evidence-Based Medicine: Literature Reviews from the National Center for Complementary and Alternative Medicine

    NIH: National Center for Complementary and Alternative Medicine (NCCAM). Evidence-Based Medicine: Literature Reviews.

    Authors' Comment: Literature reviews on various CAM modalities are provided by this NIH website. These reviews summarize what scientific evidence says about the safety and/or efficacy of certain CAM modalities. Available for free download at http://nccam.nih.gov/health/providers/litreviews.htm

3. Herbs at a Glance.

    NIH: National Center for Complementary and Alternative Medicine (NCCAM). Herbs at a Glance.

    Authors' Comment: Herbs at a Glance is a collection of fact sheets that provides information about herbs and botanicals (e.g., scientific information, common names, adverse effects, and drug interactions) that can be useful to both clinicians and patients. Available for free download at http://nccam.nih.gov/health/herbsataglance.htm

Corticosteroid-Induced Osteoporosis Prophylaxis

1. Clinician's Guide to the American College of Rheumatology 2010 Recommendations for the Prevention and Treatment of Glucocorticoid-Induced Osteoporosis.

    Authors' Comment: These are the current American College of Rheumatology recommendations for preventing and treating glucocorticoid-induced osteoporosis in adult patients. These guidelines are based on expert opinion and best available evidence and have been endorsed by the American Society for Bone and Mineral Research. Available as free download at http://www.rheumatology.org/practice/clinical/guidelines/ACR_2010_GIOP_Recomm_Clinicians_Guide.pdf

General Geriatrics Resources

1. Reconsidering medication appropriateness for patients late in life.

    Holmes HM, Hayley DC, Alexander GC, Sachs GA. Reconsidering medication appropriateness for patients late in life. Arch Intern Med. Mar 27 2006;166(6):605–609.

    Authors' Comment: This reference contains a useful framework for weighing appropriateness of medical care at the end of life for geriatric patients. Figure 2 in the reference shows the life expectancy for adults by age.

2. Geriatrics at Your Fingertips 2014

    Reuben, D. (2014). Geriatrics at Your Fingertips 2014. 16th ed. New York: American Geriatrics Society.

Authors' Comment: Geriatrics at Your Fingertips 2014 is a reference manual that covers topics such as treatment guidelines and diseases that are particularly relevant to the geriatric population. Providers can use this reference to learn more about how to properly care for the geriatric population.

Inappropriate Prescribing/ Polypharmacy

1. American Geriatrics Society. AGS Beers Criteria: Printable Beers Pocket Card.

Authors' Comment: The Beers Criteria is a catalog of drugs that can be dangerous to older adults because of age-related physiologic changes and particular pharmacologic properties of these drugs. This printable Beers pocket card, which is based on the AGS 2012 Beers Criteria, is a portable clinical tool that summarizes these drugs and can be used by providers for improving medication safety and the quality of care. Available for free download at http://www.americangeriatrics.org/files/documents/beers/PrintableBeersPocketCard.pdf

Prescription Assistance

1. The Partnership for Prescription Assistance

Authors' Comment: This website is a portal to help qualifying patients who lack prescription drug coverage acquire the medications that they need through various public or private programs that match their needs. http://www.pparx.org

References

1. Sanderson WC, Scherbov S. Measuring the speed of aging across population subgroups. PLoS One. 2014;9(5), e96289.
2. Chang AL, Wong JW, Endo JO, Norman RA. Geriatric dermatology review: major changes in skin function in older patients and their contribution to common clinical challenges. J Am Med Dir Assoc. 2013;14(10):724–30.
3. Beijer HJ, de Blaey CJ. Hospitalisations caused by adverse drug reactions (ADR): a meta-analysis of observational studies. PWS. 2002;24(2):46–54.
4. Buxton ILO, Benet LZ. Chapter 2. pharmacokinetics: The dynamics of drug absorption, distribution, metabolism, and elimination 2011.
5. Hutchison LC, Sleeper RB. Fundamentals of geriatric pharmacotherapy: an evidence-based approach. Bethesda, MD: American Society of Health-System Pharmacists; 2010. p. 463. xiv.
6. Kaestli LZ, Wasilewski-Rasca AF, Bonnabry P, Vogt-Ferrier N. Use of transdermal drug formulations in the elderly. Drugs Aging. 2008;25(4):269–80.
7. Baumgartner RN, Koehler KM, Gallagher D, Romero L, Heymsfield SB, Ross RR, et al. Epidemiology of sarcopenia among the elderly in New Mexico. Am J Epidemiol. 1998;147(8):755–63.
8. Endo JO, Wong JW, Norman RA, Chang AL. Geriatric dermatology: Part I. Geriatric pharmacology for the dermatologist. J Am Acad Dermatol. 2013;68(4):521. e1-10; quiz 31-2.
9. Turnheim K. When drug therapy gets old: pharmacokinetics and pharmacodynamics in the elderly. Exp Gerontol. 2003;38(8):843–53.
10. Sotaniemi EA, Arranto AJ, Pelkonen O, Pasanen M. Age and cytochrome P450-linked drug metabolism in humans: an analysis of 226 subjects with equal histopathologic conditions. Clin Pharmacol Ther. 1997;61(3):331–9.
11. Gonzalez Fj CMTRH. Chapter 6. drug metabolism 2011.
12. Breton G, Froissart M, Janus N, Launay-Vacher V, Berr C, Tzourio C, et al. Inappropriate drug use and mortality in community-dwelling elderly with impaired kidney function–the Three-City population-based study. Nephrol Dial Transplant. 2011;26(9):2852–9.
13. Garg AX, Papaioannou A, Ferko N, Campbell G, Clarke JA, Ray JG. Estimating the prevalence of renal insufficiency in seniors requiring long-term care. Kidney Int. 2004;65(2):649–53.
14. Flammiger A, Maibach H. Drug dosage in the elderly: dermatological drugs. Drugs Aging. 2006;23(3):203–15.
15. Rothenbacher D, Klenk J, Denkinger M, Karakas M, Nikolaus T, Peter R, et al. Prevalence and determinants of chronic kidney disease in community-dwelling elderly by various estimating equations. BMC Public Health. 2012;12:343.
16. Smith SA. Estimation of glomerular filtration rate from the serum creatinine concentration. Postgrad Med J. 1988;64(749):204–8.
17. Inker LA, Perrone RD. Assessment of kidney function. Waltham, MA: UpToDate.com; 2014. http://www.uptodate.com/contents/assessment-of-kidney-function.
18. Goldberg TH, Finkelstein MS. Difficulties in estimating glomerular filtration rate in the elderly. Arch Intern Med. 1987;147(8):1430–3.
19. Michels WM, Grootendorst DC, Verduijn M, Elliott EG, Dekker FW, Krediet RT. Performance of the

Cockcroft-Gault, MDRD, and New CKD-EPI formulas in relation to GFR, Age, and body size. Clin J Am Soc Nephrol. 2010;5(6):1003–9.

20. Walston J, Fried LP. Frailty and the older man. Med Clin North Am. 1999;83(5):1173–94.

21. Olde Rikkert MG, Rigaud AS, van Hoeyweghen RJ, de Graaf J. Geriatric syndromes: medical misnomer or progress in geriatrics? Neth J Med. 2003;61(3):83–7.

22. Tsilimingras D, Rosen AK, Berlowitz DR. Patient safety in geriatrics: a call for action. J Gerontol A: Biol Med Sci. 2003;58(9):M813–9.

23. Mitty E. Iatrogenesis, frailty, and geriatric syndromes. Geriatr Nurs (New York, NY). 2010;31(5):368–74.

24. Berry SJ, Coffey DS, Walsh PC, Ewing LL. The development of human benign prostatic hyperplasia with age. J Urol. 1984;132(3):474–9.

25. Cunningham GR, Kadmon D. Clinical manifestations and diagnostic evaluation of benign prostatic hyperplasia. Waltham, MA: UpToDate.com; 2014. http://www.uptodate.com/contents/clinical-manifestations-and-diagnostic-evaluation-of-benign-prostatic-hyperplasia?source=search_result&search=Clinical+manifestations+and+diagnostic+evaluation+of+benign+prostatic+hyperplasia&selectedTitle=1~95.

26. Coyne KS, Wein A, Nicholson S, Kvasz M, Chen CI, Milsom I. Comorbidities and personal burden of urgency urinary incontinence: a systematic review. Int J Clin Pract. 2013;67(10):1015–33.

27. Hazzard WR, Halter JB. Hazzard's geriatric medicine and gerontology. 6th ed. New York: McGraw-Hill Medical Pub. Division; 2009. xxviii, 1634 p., 12 p. of plates p.

28. Inouye SK, Westendorp RG, Saczynski JS. Delirium in elderly people. Lancet. 2014;383(9920):911–22.

29. American Geriatrics Society updated Beers Criteria for potentially inappropriate medication use in older adults. J Am Geriatrics Soc. 2012;60(4):616-31.

30. Tinetti ME. Preventing falls in elderly persons. N Engl J Med. 2003;348(1):42–9.

31. Berger TG, Steinhoff M. Pruritus in elderly patients–eruptions of senescence. Semin Cutan Med Surg. 2011;30(2):113–7.

32. Saag KG, Furst DE. Major side effects of systemic glucocorticosteroids. Waltham, MA: UpToDate.com; 2014. http://www.uptodate.com/contents/major-side-effects-of-systemic-glucocorticoids?source=search_result&search=Major+side+effects+of+systemic+glucocorticosteroids&selectedTitle=2~150.

33. Haentjens P, Magaziner J, Colon-Emeric CS, Vanderschueren D, Milisen K, Velkeniers B, et al. Meta-analysis: excess mortality after hip fracture among older women and men. Ann Intern Med. 2010;152(6):380–90.

34. van Staa TP, Leufkens HG, Cooper C. The epidemiology of corticosteroid-induced osteoporosis: a meta-analysis. Osteoporos Int. 2002;13(10):777–87.

35. Grossman JM, Gordon R, Ranganath VK, Deal C, Caplan L, Chen W, et al. American College of Rheumatology 2010 recommendations for the prevention and treatment of glucocorticoid-induced osteoporosis. Arthritis Care Res. 2010;62(11):1515–26.

36. Narum S, Westergren T, Klemp M. Corticosteroids and risk of gastrointestinal bleeding: a systematic review and meta-analysis. BMJ Open. 2014;4(5), e004587.

37. Piper JM, Ray WA, Daugherty JR, Griffin MR. Corticosteroid use and peptic ulcer disease: role of nonsteroidal anti-inflammatory drugs. Ann Intern Med. 1991;114(9):735–40.

38. Musher DM. Pneumococcal vaccination in adults. Waltham, MA: UpToDate.com; 2014. http://www.uptodate.com/contents/pneumococcal-vaccination-in-adults?source=search_result&search=Pneumococcal+vaccination+in+adults&selectedTitle=1~150.

39. Dalrymple LS, Katz R, Kestenbaum B, de Boer IH, Fried L, Sarnak MJ, et al. The risk of infection-related hospitalization with decreased kidney function. Am J Kidney Dis. 2012;59(3):356–63.

40. James MT, Quan H, Tonelli M, Manns BJ, Faris P, Laupland KB, et al. CKD and risk of hospitalization and death with pneumonia. Am J Kidney Dis. 2009;54(1):24–32.

41. Wu MY, Hsu YH, Su CL, Lin YF, Lin HW. Risk of herpes zoster in CKD: a matched-cohort study based on administrative data. Am J Kidney Dis. 2012;60(4):548–52.

42. American College of Rheumatology. Update on Herpes Zoster (Shingles) Vaccine for Autoimmune Disease Patients. 2012.

43. Bader MS. Herpes zoster: diagnostic, therapeutic, and preventive approaches. Postgrad Med. 2013;125(5):78–91.

44. Saag KG, Koehnke R, Caldwell JR, Brasington R, Burmeister LF, Zimmerman B, et al. Low dose long-term corticosteroid therapy in rheumatoid arthritis: an analysis of serious adverse events. Am J Med. 1994;96(2):115–23.

45. Noninfluenza vaccination coverage among adults—United States, 2011. MMWR Morbidity and mortality weekly report. 2013;62(4):66-72.

46. Rubin LG, Levin MJ, Ljungman P, Davies EG, Avery R, Tomblyn M, et al. 2013 IDSA clinical practice guideline for vaccination of the immuno-compromised host. Clin Infect Dis. 2014;58(3):e44–100.

47. Kunisaki KM, Janoff EN. Influenza in immunosuppressed populations: a review of infection frequency, morbidity, mortality, and vaccine responses. Lancet Infect Dis. 2009;9(8):493–504.

48. Mansharamani NG, Garland R, Delaney D, Koziel H. Management and outcome patterns for adult Pneumocystis carinii pneumonia, 1985 to 1995: comparison of HIV-associated cases to other immunocompromised states. Chest. 2000;118(3):704–11.

49. Suryaprasad A, Stone JH. When is it safe to stop Pneumocystis jiroveci pneumonia prophylaxis?

Insights from three cases complicating autoimmune diseases. Arthritis Rheum. 2008;59(7):1034–9.

50. Thomas Jr CF, Limper AH. Pneumocystis pneumonia. N Engl J Med. 2004;350(24):2487–98.

51. Limper AH, Knox KS, Sarosi GA, Ampel NM, Bennett JE, Catanzaro A, et al. An official American thoracic society statement: treatment of fungal infections in adult pulmonary and critical care patients. Am J Respir Crit Care Med. 2011;183(1):96–128.

52. Roblot F, Le Moal G, Kauffmann-Lacroix C, Bastides F, Boutoille D, Verdon R, et al. Pneumocystis Jirovecii pneumonia in HIV-negative patients: a prospective study with focus on immunosuppressive drugs and markers of immune impairment. Scand J Infect Dis. 2014;46(3):210–4.

53. Bodro M, Paterson DL. Has the time come for routine trimethoprim-sulfamethoxazole prophylaxis in patients taking biologic therapies? Clin Infect Dis. 2013;56(11):1621–8.

54. Green H, Paul M, Vidal L, Leibovici L. Prophylaxis of Pneumocystis pneumonia in immunocompromised non-HIV-infected patients: systematic review and meta-analysis of randomized controlled trials. Mayo Clin Proc. 2007;82(9):1052–9.

55. Saladi RN, Persaud AN. The causes of skin cancer: a comprehensive review. Drugs Today. 2005;41(1): 37–53. Barcelona, Spain : 1998.

56. Karagas MR, Cushing Jr GL, Greenberg ER, Mott LA, Spencer SK, Nierenberg DW. Non-melanoma skin cancers and glucocorticoid therapy. Br J Cancer. 2001;85(5):683–6.

57. Targownik LE, Bernstein CN. Infectious and malignant complications of TNF inhibitor therapy in IBD. Am J Gastroenterol. 2013;108(12):1835–42. quiz 43.

58. Williams JR. The world medical association medical ethics manual. The World Medical Association. 2nd ed. Ferney-Voltaire Cedex: The World Medical Association; 2009.

59. Appelbaum PS, Grisso T. Assessing patients' capacities to consent to treatment. N Engl J Med. 1988; 319(25):1635–8.

60. Sessums LL, Zembrzuska H, Jackson JL. Does this patient have medical decision-making capacity? JAMA. 2011;306(4):420–7.

61. Fontanella D, Grant-Kels JM, Patel T, Norman R. Ethical issues in geriatric dermatology. Clin Dermatol. 2012;30(5):511–5.

62. Khalil H. Prescribing for the elderly: ethical considerations. Aust J Prim Health. 2011;17(1):2–3.

63. Le Couteur DG, Ford GA, McLachlan AJ. Evidence, ethics and medication management in older people. J Pharm Res. 2010;40(2):4.

64. Holmes HM, Hayley DC, Alexander GC, Sachs GA. Reconsidering medication appropriateness for patients late in life. Arch Intern Med. 2006;166(6): 605–9.

65. Zulman DM, Sussman JB, Chen X, Cigolle CT, Blaum CS, Hayward RA. Examining the evidence: a systematic review of the inclusion and analysis of older adults in randomized controlled trials. J Gen Intern Med. 2011;26(7):783–90.

66. Linnebur SA, O'Connell MB, Wessell AM, McCord AD, Kennedy DH, DeMaagd G, et al. Pharmacy practice, research, education, and advocacy for older adults. Pharmacotherapy. 2005;25(10):1396–430.

67. Dalleur O, Spinewine A, Henrard S, Losseau C, Speybroeck N, Boland B. Inappropriate prescribing and related hospital admissions in frail older persons according to the STOPP and START criteria. Drugs Aging. 2012;29(10):829–37.

68. Rocchiccioli JT, Sanford J, Caplinger B. Polymedicine and aging—Enhancing older adult care through advanced practitioners. J Gerontol Nurs. 2007;33(7):19–24.

69. Gupta M, Agarwal M. Understanding medication errors in the elderly. N Z Med J. 2013;126(1385): 62–70.

70. Beers MH. Explicit criteria for determining potentially inappropriate medication use by the elderly— An update. Arch Intern Med. 1997;157(14):1531–6.

71. Rochon PA. Drug prescribing for older adults. Waltham, MA: UpToDate.com; 2014. p. 33. http:// www.uptodate.com/contents/drug-prescribing-for-older-adults?source=search_result&search=Drug+P rescribing+for+Older+Adults&selectedTi tle=1~150.

72. Opondo D, Eslami S, Visscher S, de Rooij SE, Verheij R, Korevaar JC, et al. Inappropriateness of medication prescriptions to elderly patients in the primary care setting: a systematic review. PLoS One. 2012;7(8):e43617.

73. Stockl KM, Le L, Zhang S, Harada AS. Clinical and economic outcomes associated with potentially inappropriate prescribing in the elderly. Am J Manag Care. 2010;16(1):e1–10.

74. Goldstein R, Thompson FE, McKendry RJ. Diagnostic and predictive value of the lupus band test in undifferentiated connective tissue disease. A followup study. J Rheumatol. 1985;12(6):1093–6.

75. Gupta MA, Gupta AK, Fink NH. Polypharmacy in dermatology: analysis of a nationally representative sample of 46,273 dermatology patient visits in the United States from 1995 to 2009. Skinmed. 2013; 11(5):273–80.

76. Viktil KK, Blix HS, Moger TA, Reikvam A. Polypharmacy as commonly defined is an indicator of limited value in the assessment of drug-related problems. Br J Clin Pharmacol. 2007;63(2):187–95.

77. Field TS, Gurwitz JH, Avorn J, McCormick D, Jain S, Eckler M, et al. Risk factors for adverse drug events among nursing home residents. Arch Intern Med. 2001;161(13):1629–34.

78. Tinetti ME, Bogardus ST, Agostini JV. Potential pitfalls of disease-specific guidelines for patients with multiple conditions. N Engl J Med. 2004;351(27): 2870–4.

79. Rochon PA, Gurwitz JH. Optimising drug treatment for elderly people: the prescribing cascade. Br Med J. 1997;315(7115):1096–9.

80. Weng MC, Tsai CF, Sheu KL, Lee YT, Lee HC, Tzeng SL, et al. The impact of number of drugs prescribed on the risk of potentially inappropriate

medication among outpatient older adults with chronic diseases. Qjm-An Int J Med. 2013;106(11): 1009–15.

81. Ganeva M, Gancheva T, Troeva J, Kiriyak N, Hristakieva E. Clinical relevance of drug-drug interactions in hospitalized dermatology patients. Adv Clin Exp Med. 2013;22(4):555–63.

82. Cherubini A, Corsonello A, Lattanzio F. Underprescription of beneficial medicines in older people: causes, consequences and prevention. Drugs Aging. 2012;29(6):463–75.

83. Kuijpers MA, van Marum RJ, Egberts AC, Jansen PA, Group OS. Relationship between polypharmacy and underprescribing. Br J Clin Pharmacol. 2008; 65(1):130–3.

84. Cherubini A, Ruggiero C, Gasperini B, Dell'Aquila G, Cupido MG, Zampi E, et al. The prevention of adverse drug reactions in older subjects. Curr Drug Metab. 2011;12(7):652–7.

85. Tulner LR, van Campen J, Frankfort SV, Koks CHW, Beijnen JH, Brandjes DPM, et al. Changes in undertreatment after comprehensive geriatric assessment an observational study. Drugs Aging. 2010;27(10): 831–43.

86. Osterberg L, Blaschke T. Drug therapy—adherence to medication. N Engl J Med. 2005;353(5):487–97.

87. Caskie GIL, Willis SL, Schaie KW, Zanjani FAK. Congruence of medication information from a brown bag data collection and pharmacy records: Findings from the Seattle Longitudinal Study. Exp Aging Res. 2006;32(1):79–103.

88. Richmond NA, Lamel SA, Braun LR, Vivas AC, Cucalon J, Block SG, et al. Primary nonadherence (failure to obtain prescribed medicines) among dermatology patients. J Am Acad Dermatol. 2014;70(1): 201–3.

89. Gurwitz JH, Field TS, Harrold LR, Rothschild J, Debellis K, Seger AC, et al. Incidence and preventability of adverse drug events among older persons in the ambulatory setting. JAMA. 2003;289(9):1107–16.

90. Chiatti C, Bustacchini S, Furneri G, Mantovani L, Cristiani M, Misuraca C, et al. The economic burden of inappropriate drug prescribing, lack of adherence and compliance, adverse drug events in older people: a systematic review. Drug Saf. 2012;35 Suppl 1:73–87.

91. Balkrishnan R, Rajagopalan R, Camacho FT, Huston SA, Murray FT, Anderson RT. Predictors of medication adherence and associated health care costs in an older population with type 2 diabetes mellitus: a longitudinal cohort study. Clin Ther. 2003;25(11):2958–71.

92. Field TS, Mazor KM, Briesacher B, Debellis KR, Gurwitz JH. Adverse drug events resulting from patient errors in older adults. J Am Geriatr Soc. 2007;55(2):271–6.

93. Smith M, Bailey T. Identifying solutions to medication adherence in the visually impaired elderly. Consult Pharm. 2014;29(2):131–4.

94. Wilson IB, Schoen C, Neuman P, Strollo MK, Rogers WH, Chang H, et al. Physician-patient communication about prescription medication nonadherence: A 50-state study of America's seniors. J Gen Intern Med. 2007;22(1):6–12.

95. Pasina L, Brucato AL, Falcone C, Cucchi E, Bresciani A, Sottocorno M, et al. Medication Nonadherence among elderly patients newly discharged and receiving polypharmacy. Drugs Aging. 2014; 31(4):283–9.

96. Modig S, Kristensson J, Troein M, Brorsson A, Midlov P. Frail elderly patients' experiences of information on medication. A qualitative study. BMC Geriatr. 2012;12:46.

97. National Center for Complementary and Alternative Medicine (NCCAM). Complementary, Alternative, or Integrative Health: What's In a Name? Bethesda, MDMay 2013 [May 6, 2014]. Available from: http://nccam.nih.gov/health/whatiscam.

98. Ernst E. Adverse effects of herbal drugs in dermatology. Br J Dermatol. 2000;143(5):923–9.

99. Kaufman DW, Kelly JP, Rosenberg L, Anderson TE, Mitchell AA. Recent patterns of medication use in the ambulatory adult population of the United States— The Slone survey. JAMA. 2002;287(3):337–44.

100. Kelly JP, Kaufman DW, Kelley K, Rosenberg L, Anderson TE, Mitchell AA. Recent trends in use of herbal and other natural products. Arch Intern Med. 2005;165(3):281–6.

101. Qato DM, Alexander GC, Conti RM, Johnson M, Schumm P, Lindau ST. Use of prescription and over-the-counter medications and dietary supplements among older adults in the United States. JAMA. 2008;300(24):2867–78.

102. Fuhrmann T, Smith N, Tausk F. Use of complementary and alternative medicine among adults with skin disease: Updated results from a national survey. J Am Acad Dermatol. 2010;63(6):1000–5.

103. Bishop FL, Yardley L, Lewith GT. A systematic review of beliefs involved in the use of complementary and alternative medicine. J Health Psychol. 2007;12(6):851–67.

104. Cheung CK, Wyman JF, Halcon LL. Use of complementary and alternative therapies in community-dwelling older adults. J Altern Complement Med (New York, NY). 2007;13(9):997–1006.

105. Arcury TA, Bell RA, Altizer KP, Grzywacz JG, Sandberg JC, Quandt SA. Attitudes of older adults regarding disclosure of complementary therapy use to physicians. J Appl Gerontol. 2013;32(5):627–45.

106. Faith J, Thorburn S, Tippens KM. Examining CAM use disclosure using the behavioral model of health services use. Complement Ther Med. 2013;21(5):501–8.

107. Mechanick JI, Brett EM, Chausmer AB, Dickey RA, Wallach S. American Association of Clinical Endocrinologists medical guidelines for the clinical use of dietary supplements and nutraceuticals. Endocr Pract. 2003;9(5):417–70.

108. Ernst E. The usage of complementary therapies by dermatological patients: a systematic review. Br J Dermatol. 2000;142(5):857–61.

109. Koo J, Arain S. Traditional Chinese medicine for the treatment of dermatologic disorders. Arch Dermatol. 1998;134(11):1388–93.

110. McAleer MA, Powell FC. Complementary and alternative medicine usage in rosacea. Br J Dermatol. 2008;158(5):1139–41.

111. Bielory L. Complementary and alternative interventions in asthma, allergy, and immunology. Ann Allergy Asthma Immunol. 2004;93(2):S45–54.

112. Niggemann B, Gruber C. Side-effects of complementary and alternative medicine. Allergy. 2003;58(8):707–16.

113. Wold RS, Lopez ST, Yau CL, Butler LM, Pareo-Tubbeh SL, Waters DL, et al. Increasing trends in elderly persons' use of nonvitamin, nonmineral dietary supplements and concurrent use of medications. J Am Diet Assoc. 2005;105(1):54–63.

114. Fugh-Berman A. Herb-drug interactions. Lancet. 2000;355(9198):134–8.

115. Gupta SK, Kaleekal T, Joshi S. Misuse of corticosteroids in some of the drugs dispensed as preparations from alternative systems of medicine in India. Pharmacoepidemiol Drug Saf. 2000;9(7):599–602.

116. Keane FM, Munn SE, du Vivier AWP, Higgins EM, Taylor NF. Analysis of Chinese herbal creams prescribed for dermatological conditions (Reprinted from BMJ, vol 318, pg 563-4, 1999). West J Med. 1999;170(5):257–9.

117. Spinewine A, Schmader KE, Barber N, Hughes C, Lapane KL, Swine C, et al. Appropriate prescribing in elderly people: how well can it be measured and optimised? Lancet. 2007;370(9582):173–84.

118. Steinman MA, Hanlon JT. Managing medications in clinically complex elders: "There's got to be a happy medium". JAMA. 2010;304(14):1592–601.

119. Steinman MA, Handler SM, Gurwitz JH, Schiff GD, Covinsky KE. Beyond the prescription: medication monitoring and adverse drug events in older adults. J Am Geriatr Soc. 2011;59(8):1513–20.

120. Endo J, Jacobsen K. Medication reconciliation in Wisconsin: insights from a local initiative. WMJ. 2006;105(8):42–4.

121. Bain KT, Holmes HM, Beers MH, Maio V, Handler SM, Pauker SG. Discontinuing medications: a novel approach for revising the prescribing stage of the medication-use process. J Am Geriatr Soc. 2008;56(10):1946–52.

122. Green CB, Stratman EJ. Prevent rather than treat postherpetic neuralgia by prescribing gabapentin earlier in patients with herpes zoster: comment on "incidence of postherpetic neuralgia after combination treatment with gabapentin and valacyclovir in patients with acute herpes zoster". Arch Dermatol. 2011;147(8):908.

123. Labbate LA. Drugs for the treatment of depression. Handbook of psychiatric drug therapy. 6th ed. Philadelphia, PA: Wolters Kluwer Health; 2010. p. xiv, 304.

124. Prakash AV, Davis MD. Contact dermatitis in older adults: a review of the literature. Am J Clin Dermatol. 2010;11(6):373–81.

125. Zirwas MJ, Stechschulte SA. Moisturizer allergy: diagnosis and management. J Clin Aesthet Dermatol. 2008;1(4):38–44.

126. Coopman S, Degreef H, Dooms-Goossens A. Identification of cross-reaction patterns in allergic contact dermatitis from topical corticosteroids. Br J Dermatol. 1989;121(1):27–34.

127. Dermatology. 2e ed. Bolognia JL, Jorizzo JL, Rapini RP, editors. St. Louis, MO: Elsevier; 2008.

128. Al Jasser M, Mebuke N, de Gannes GC. Propylene glycol: an often unrecognized cause of allergic contact dermatitis in patients using topical corticosteroids. Skin Ther Lett. 2011;16(5):5–7.

129. Harris K, Curtis J, Larsen B, Calder S, Duffy K, Bowen G, et al. Opioid pain medication use after dermatologic surgery: A prospective observational study of 212 dermatologic surgery patients. JAMA Dermatol. 2013;149(3):317–21.

130. Bronaugh RL, Maibach HI. Percutaneous absorption: drugs–cosmetics–mechanisms–methodology. 3rd ed. New York, NY: Marcel Dekker; 1999.

131. Goldstein B, Goldstein AO. General principles of dermatologic therapy and topical corticosteroid use. Waltham, MA: UpToDate.com; 2013. http://www.uptodate.com/contents/general-principles-of-dermatologic-therapy-and-topical-corticosteroid-use?source=search_result&search=General+principles+of+dermatologic+therapy+and+topical+corticosteroid+use&selectedTitle=1~150.

132. Kalichman L, Hernandez-Molina G. Hand osteoarthritis: an epidemiological perspective. Semin Arthritis Rheum. 2010;39(6):465–76.

133. Nikolaus T, Kruse W, Bach M, Specht-Leible N, Oster P, Schlierf G. Elderly patients' problems with medication. An in-hospital and follow-up study. Eur J Clin Pharmacol. 1996;49(4):255–9.

134. Murray MD, Morrow DG, Weiner M, Clark DO, Tu W, Deer MM, et al. A conceptual framework to study medication adherence in older adults. Am J Geriatr Pharmacother. 2004;2(1):36–43.

135. Sudore RL, Schillinger D. Interventions to improve care for patients with limited health literacy. JCOM. 2009;16(1):20–9.

136. Ryan R, Santesso N, Lowe D, Hill S, Grimshaw J, Prictor M, et al. Interventions to improve safe and effective medicines use by consumers: an overview of systematic reviews. Cochrane Database Syst Rev. 2014;4, CD007768.

137. Garfinkel D, Mangin D. Feasibility study of a systematic approach for discontinuation of multiple medications in older adults: addressing polypharmacy. Arch Intern Med. 2010;170(18):1648–54.

138. Topinkova E, Baeyens JP, Michel JP, Lang PO. Evidence-based strategies for the optimization of pharmacotherapy in older people. Drugs Aging. 2012;29(6):477–94.

139. Heaton E, Levender MM, Feldman SR. Timing of office visits can be a powerful tool to improve adherence in the treatment of dermatologic conditions. J Dermatolog Treat. 2013;24(2):82–8.

140. Tan X, Feldman SR, Chang JW, Balkrishnan R. Topical drug delivery systems in dermatology: a review of patient adherence issues. Expert Opin Drug Deliv. 2012;9(10):1263–71.

Pruritus in Older Patients

Kevin Chun-Kai Wang

> Many persons, of both sexes, so incessantly tormented with a violent and universal itching, that they were rendered uncomfortable for the remainder of life.—Robert Willan, 1809

Scope of Itch in the Elderly

While it is often said that pruritus (itching), best defined as an unpleasant sensation that leads to a desire to scratch, is the most frequent symptom in dermatology [1] there are surprisingly few studies about the prevalence or incidence of pruritus in particular diseases or in specific patient populations. The elderly are believed to be particularly prone to pruritus, especially chronic pruritus—the regression in the integrity of the human integumentary system over time is well documented, and include loss of skin hydration, a proinflammatory immune system [2], loss of collagen, and a higher incidence of dry skin secondary to reduction in the concentration of epidermal lipids and sweat/sebum production [3].

Estimates of prevalence range between 11.5 and 41 % [4, 5]. In fact, itch is the most common dermatologic complaint in people over the age of 65 years [5–9]; xerosis was a close second in a study from the 1990s [10], with most dermatologists recognizing dry skin as the most common cause of pruritus in the elderly [10]. Interestingly, the term "senile pruritus" or "Willan's itch" was introduced and widely used in the medical literature to describe chronic pruritus of unknown origin in old-age individuals [11, 12]. Perhaps even more telling, is the comment that "senile pruritus" being synonymous with "the common complaint of unexplained itching in the elderly," and that it is a "diagnosis of exclusion" [11]. Regrettably, the cause(s) of senile pruritus remain incompletely understood now as it had been in 1809.

The elderly in the USA represent the fastest growing segment of the population, with the oldest group (>85 years) having had the highest percentage growth over the past two decades; an even sharper growth is expected after 2030 when baby boomers reach this age [13]. This rapid demographic shift has created challenges both to the health care system and to society at large. Curiously, there appears to be no general consensus in the medical literature as to what constitute the "elderly"—i.e., there is no precise cut-off age—furthermore, it is unclear what clinical presentations of itch are to be expected in these patient populations [6, 14]. There is no question that the inevitable increase in itching amongst the elderly patient population represents a growing challenge due to the changing demographic distribution. This burden of disease in the elderly is almost certainly underestimated, based on the available data [14].

K.C.-K. Wang, M.D., Ph.D. (✉)
Assistant Professor, Department of Dermatology, Stanford University School of Medicine, 269 Campus Drive CCSR 2115A, Stanford, CA 94305, USA
e-mail: kevwang@stanford.edu

© Springer International Publishing Switzerland 2015
A.L.S. Chang (ed.), *Advances in Geriatric Dermatology*, DOI 10.1007/978-3-319-18380-0_2

Many conditions prevalent in the elderly contribute to itching. Itching can occur in isolation or associated with a primary skin disease, a systemic disorder (chronic renal and liver insufficiency), or it may have multifactorial or idiopathic causes [10]. In addition, polypharmacy is common owing to the high frequency of chronic diseases present in this population, and many systemic and topical drugs can induce pruritus [15]. Furthermore, itch may be indicative of an underlying malignancy such as lymphoma, solid tumors, or myelodysplastic syndromes.

Classic Clinical Studies Related to Itch in the Elderly

All humans experience pruritus in the course of their lifetime. It can be an important lead symptom in many systemic disorders, the most common being chronic renal insufficiency, cholestatic liver disease, diabetes, and lymphoma [1, 14, 16]. In addition, pruritus often has a profound impact on quality of life through disturbances related to sleep, attention, and sexual function [16]. Maladaptive sleep patterns and mood disturbances including anxiety and depression are common in pruritic patients, and may exacerbate the itching [16]. In fact, a recent study demonstrated that chronic itch to be as debilitating as chronic pain [17]. Perhaps not surprisingly, chronic pruritus is an enormous burden to society through treatment-related costs, which is especially large as a result of the high rate of therapeutic failure in these patients [18]. To complicate matters, clinical experience indicates that patients frequently do not consult a physician for acute itch, but more often do for chronic itch (defined as itch lasting longer than 6 weeks) [1]. Furthermore, most of the studies in the literature refer to specific diseases or patient groups, which complicates the comparability and validity of the existing studies.

Population-based prevalence studies of pruritus in the geriatric population are lacking. Most studies to date are limited by small sample sizes, selection bias, and divergent study end-points. For example, a study in the 1980s that focused on skin problems in the elderly (ages 50–91 years) found that pruritus was the most frequent complaint, affecting nearly one-third of nursing home patients [6]. Another study with a much larger cohort of patients found that itch ranked first amongst the distribution of skin diseases (11.5 %), affecting more women than men, with the highest prevalence in patients 85 years or older (19.5 %); interestingly, itch was always found to be in the top five most frequent diagnoses regardless of season, especially during winter and autumn [5]. In another study, pruritic diseases and xerosis were the most common complaints (41 % and 39 %, respectively) [4]. These studies highlight the need for more well-designed epidemiological research in order to establish an evidence base for the claim that pruritus is more frequent in the elderly.

Drugs and Pruritus

Pruritus is commonly listed as a medication complication, but the prevalence of drug-induced pruritus has not been well-studied to date. One classic large epidemiological study from the 1980s showed that, among hospitalized patients, pruritus without concomitant skin lesions accounted for approximately 5 % of adverse reactions after drug intake [19]. Unfortunately, these data are difficult to extrapolate to drugs that are prescribed in outpatient clinics, as only inpatients were analyzed. There is also scant data regarding the prevalence of drug-induced pruritus in the elderly population—a Turkish study estimated the frequency to be between 1.3 and 1.6 % of the patients over 65 years old [5]. The role of topical and systemic medications in pruritus in the elderly remains poorly understood.

The most important drugs that have been implicated to be major contributors to itch in the elderly from a large case–control study included cardiac (diuretics, angiotensin-converting enzyme inhibitors, calcium channel blockers, hypolipidemic drugs), salicylates, and chemotherapeutic agents [20]. Interestingly, the pathogenesis of drug-induced pruritus differs depending upon the causative agent—for example, pruritus may be caused by drug-induced skin eruptions, or it may be due to a number of alternative mechanisms including cholestatic liver injury, phototoxicity, xerosis, drug and/or drug metabolite deposition in the skin, or neuropathic dysregulation. A handful of medications have been reported to cause pruritus with no or only a transient eruption, including angiotensin-converting enzyme inhibitors, statins, salicylates, chloroquine, and calcium channel blockers [18, 21].

Unfortunately, the underlying mechanism is often unknown or never elucidated [15, 21]. However, treatment of the pruritus should not be delayed while awaiting a response from medication cessation [15].

Eruption of Senescence

Aging affects three principal components involved in the generation of pruritus—the immune system, the epidermal barrier, and the nervous system.

The age-associated decline in systemic immunity, referred to as "immunosenescense" [22, 23], is characterized by a decrease in cell-mediated immune function as well as by reduced humoral immune responses. Age-dependent defects in T- and B-cell function coexist with age-related changes within the innate immune system [23], including a higher level of proinflammatory activity. This significant T and B cell dysregulation can result in an "allergic" phenotype in some patients, with a change towards Type 2 dominance (Th2) [24]. The proinflammatory state is believed to develop as a result of loss of naïve T cells.

Aging also significant alters the epidermal barrier. The increased in surface pH of the epidermis manifests initially as a reduced rate of barrier repair which in turn results in loss of barrier maintenance capabilities and decrease in epidermal hydration [2]. Xerosis is consequently an inevitable outcome in the elderly population [25]. An impaired barrier can then lead subsequently to increased risk for the development of contact dermatitis, due to penetration of potential antigens into the epidermis, and increased release of proinflammatory cytokines [2]. This is perhaps most aptly illustrated in atopic dermatitis, where the relationship and interplay between defective epidermal barrier and cutaneous inflammation are immediately evident.

Finally, the elderly are frequently afflicted with degenerative diseases of the spine. The degenerative lesion can result in impingements on sensory nerves as they exit the spinal cord, and is the primary cause of the underlying pruritus. Brachioradial pruritus (BRP) and notalgia paresthetica (NP) are two conditions with this presumed pathogenesis [26]. In addition, in rare cases, neurodegenerative disease of the central nervous system may produce itching [2]. These patients will often present with secondary morphologies of lichenification, such as lichen simplex chronicus, prurigo nodularis (Fig. 1), and macular amyloid, and invariably complain of

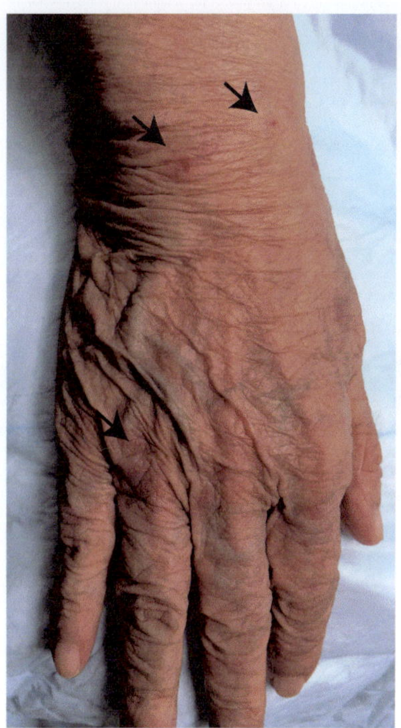

Fig. 1 Prurigo Nodularis. Prurigo nodularis nodules or papules are discrete, scaly, hyperpigmented or purpuric, firm lesions (arrows) that are a few millimeters in diameter. Some lesions have a characteristic raised warty surface. Earlier lesions may start as smaller nondescript red "bumps." Nodules and papules occur on the extensor surfaces of the arm, legs, and trunk. Prurigo nodularis lesions may show signs of excoriation with flat, umbilicated, or crusted top. The nodule pattern may be follicular. The skin in between the nodules is often dry

both itching and additional forms of dysesthesia (numbness, burning, or tingling sensations). The typical topical anti-inflammatories are ineffective, and some cases respond only to application of ice [2]. As described above, the most common clinical diagnoses were brachioradial pruritus and notalgia paresthetica [27, 28]. Occasionally patients complain of more diffuse pruritus related to a generalized neuropathy; diabetic neuropathy with generalized truncal pruritus is one such example [29].

A useful way to tie all three aspects together is to think about the primary morphology that the patient presents. Underlying neurological diseases should always be part of the differential. Not infrequently in these patients, multiple types of lesions coexist, or appear over time (Fig. 2). For instance, a patient may present initially with lichenified lesions of atopic dermatitis (suggestive of a barrier defect), only to represent weeks to months later with a widespread papular eruption (evidence of a primary immunological phenomenon). By considering all of these discrete morphologies as a consequence of an "eruption of senescence," one can apply understanding of the physiological changes of aging to better elucidate the factors responsible for each of the specific morphologic patterns [2].

General Measures for Treatments of Itch in Elderly Patients

As discussed previously, pruritus in the elderly can be caused by a multitude of factors and physiological changes that occur with aging, including impaired skin barrier function, immunosenescence, neuropathies, and polypharmacy [2]. Therefore, the identification of one potential cause for pruritus does not eliminate the need to complete a full evaluation. Unfortunately, little evidence supports pruritus treatment, limiting therapeutic possibilities and resulting in challenging management problems. Thus, it is essential to recognize the profound effect pruritus can have on a patient's function and quality of life, as part of the approach to treatment. As with other symptoms in the geriatric population, pruritus evaluation requires integration and consideration of all of the patient's medical conditions [21]. Furthermore, management of pruritus in the elderly can be challenging because of additional physical and/or cognitive limitations. Elderly patients are frequently unable to apply topical treatments effectively on their own, and medication compliance becomes a major issue. In addition, comorbid conditions and polypharmacy increase the risk of adverse drug reactions,

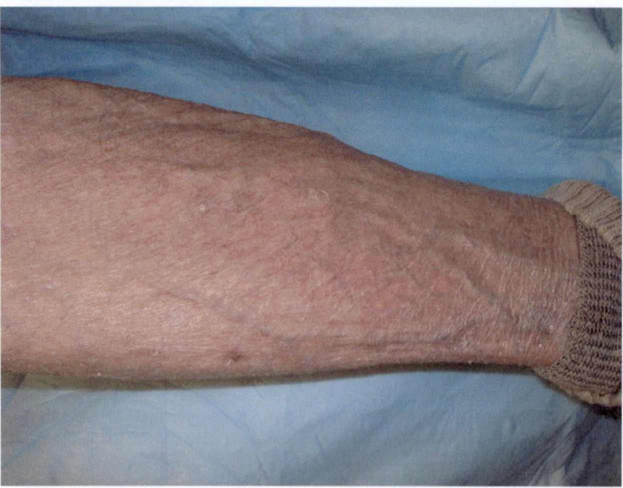

Fig. 2 Representative view of polymorphic eruption. The presence of scattered eroded erythematous papules with linear urticarial plaques is typical of eruptions of senescence. Note the background xerosis and hyperpigmented patches consistent with prior inflammatory dermatosis

Table 1 Summary of current treatment options for itching in the elderly

Type of treatment	Examples	Comments
Barrier Repair (Dry skin care)	Emollients	Older patients with musculoskeletal or visual problems may experience difficulties with application; may require significant caregiver assistance
Topical corticosteroids	Triamcinolone Hydrocortisone	Older patients with musculoskeletal or visual problems may experience difficulties with application; may require significant caregiver assistance; may only be effective in primarily inflammatory conditions
Systemic (oral) antihistamines	Sedating: hydroxyzine, diphenhydramine, doxepin Nonsedating: cetirizine, loratidine	Avoid in elderly due to side effects of somnolence, anticholinergic effects, risk of falls
Capsaicinoids	Capsaicin cream	Desensitizes sensory nerve fibers; application connected with burning sensations during first days of use
Ultraviolet therapy	Narrowband	Older patient must be able to stand stably in the booths; good choice for patients with multiple underlying etiologies for itching and/or polypharmacy
Neuromodulators	Antileptics: gabapentin, pregabalin Antidepressants: paroxetine or fluvoxamine	Most effective in patients with neuropathic pruritus, pruritus of chronic renal failure, cholestatic pruritus
Opiate receptor antagonist or agonists	μ-opiate receptor blockade: naltrexone κ-opiate receptor activation: nalfurafine	Most effective in patients with liver or kidney disease; side effects often limits practicality of use in elderly

especially with systemic therapy. Any treatment plan must take into consideration the patient's general health, living situation, severity of symptoms, and the adverse effects of available treatment(s) [21, 30]. Because the immunosenescence that drives the pruritus is not reversible, long-term treatment with a combination of modalities is often required. Table 1 summarizes the most commonly employed therapeutic options in these patients.

Topical immunomodulators, including medium to ultrapotent strength topical corticosteroids and calcineurin inhibitors, are reasonable first-line agents for elderly patients with moderate-to-severe pruritus that is secondary to localized inflammatory skin processes. The topical therapies should always be instituted with concurrent aggressive emollient use and gentle skin care to improve skin barrier function. Because of the increased fragility of senescent skin, prolonged topical corticosteroid use should be avoided to prevent development of atrophy.

Antihistamines are a popular adjunct medication often used as antipruritic agents, because of the presumed benefit of sedation; yet there is limited evidence with respect to their efficacy in treating chronic pruritus in elderly patients—in fact, there is only one small randomized trial from the early 1980s with oxatomide, a first-generation antihistamine, where it was shown to improve both the duration and severity of itching [31]. In fact, antihistamine use in the older population is generally not recommended due to the anticholinergic effects (confusion, constipation, and dry mouth) [32]. Furthermore, there is little evidence that standard second-generation nonsedating antihistamines are effective in the management of pruritus in elderly patients [16]. Neuromodulatory agents such as gabapentin may be tried instead, dosed according to the underlying state and response of each patient [21].

UV-based therapy (phototherapy and photochemotherapy) is an alternative treatment modality that can be effective for certain pruritic conditions—for example, dermatoses with an atopic dermatitis-like component, pruritus associated with renal failure, and even pruritus of unclear etiology [21]. Phototherapy, including narrowband or broadband UVB, or less often UVA, is widely used in patients of all ages with chronic pruritus [33], and has been shown to be effective in treating a variety of pruritic conditions that afflict elderly patients, including pruritus due to atopic dermatitis, renal failure, polycythemia vera, chronic liver disease, and Hodgkin's lymphoma [34]. It has wide cutaneous anti-inflammatory activities, and can offer relief without many of the adverse effects and risks of systemic immunosuppressive medications. Its efficacy has also been demonstrated in some randomized controlled trials [34–36]. Areas of long-term sun exposure (head and neck, dorsal hands) can be protected to avoid increasing skin cancer risk in these regions.

For patients with primary lesions, medications, contactants, and photosensitivity must be considered as causal or coexistent factors that are contributing to the pruritus. For the majority of these patients, barrier failure is often present, and a "soak and smear" approach to initiate treatment is often very effective. Soaking in a warm tub for 15 min and applying a high-potency topical steroid diluted in a heavy moisturizer such as petrolatum, onto the wet skin followed by an occlusion (with a suit or wet wraps) can be quite effective [2]. Antihistamines can be used with caution to complement the topical steroids, and phototherapy can be considered in refractory cases. If the dermatitis and pruritus remain chronic and treatment-resistant, low-dose immunosuppressive agents may be useful. Methotrexate, azathioprine, or mycophenolate mofetil can all be effective systemic medications, with the agent used dependent upon the patient's risk profile, comorbidities, and at times, medication availability [2, 33]. Occasionally, after barrier repair has been accomplished via aggressive topical regimens, and the inflammatory reaction calms, the systemic immunosuppressive(s) can then be removed gradually and the patient maintained with topical treatment or phototherapy.

In the patient with generalized pruritus and secondary skin morphologies only, a primarily neuropathic process of the peripheral or central nervous system should be sought. Neurally acting antipruritic agents such as gabapentin, duloxetine, and mirtazepine alone or in combination can be effective [2, 21, 33]. Neurologists and physical medicine physicians are often useful in aiding the evaluation of such patients.

Research Gaps, Ongoing Clinical Trials

In recent years, pruritus has garnered more attention and is now appreciated as an important symptom that can dramatically reduce quality of life in patients [9]. Unfortunately, the pathophysiology of pruritus is only partially understood. The optimal evaluation strategy with respect to yield and cost-effectiveness has not been determined, and data from randomized, controlled trials of various pharmacologic and nonpharmacologic treatments for chronic pruritus are scarce. It is clear that more high-quality research is needed in order to be able to assess the burden of pruritus in specific diseases and patient populations. The empirical basis for an assessment in the general population is growing but replications of the available findings in specific patient groups would be desirable. Nevertheless, the recent population-based studies have revealed various new insights regarding the epidemiological underpinnings of chronic pruritus (e.g., prevalence, incidence, and determinants).

In daily clinical practice, consideration of coexisting disease and overlapping symptoms across diseases may help in the attribution of the cause of pruritus. The role of mixed etiologies has rarely been studied. This is of growing importance, especially in elderly individuals who are more likely to suffer from several diseases (multi-morbidity) and regularly require medication(s). Taking this multi-morbidity into account will, however, make the design of epidemiological research attempting to quantify the frequency of pruritus in patient populations much more complex.

Pruritus, like pain, is a stimulus that cannot be measured directly. Currently, most ongoing clinical studies are concentrated on methods of pruritus assessment. Despite many issues that have already been answered, there are still a number of problems remain—for example, development of a new, widely accepted itch questionnaire is essential to provide a valid instrument for multiple studies, to enable better comparisons of various pruritus subtypes and different treatment strategies. Chronic pruritus poses a significant threat to overall quality of life (QoL). A recent survey of patients with chronic pruritus and those with chronic pain (mean age of participants was 55 years), which utilized directly elicited health utility scores, demonstrated that chronic pruritus has an impact comparable to that of chronic pain on QoL [17], underscoring the significant burden of disease with which chronic itch patients suffer. In fact, studies in patients with uremic pruritus have suggested that itch, via its impact on sleep, not only affects morbidity, but increases mortality [37].

The next steps in chronic pruritus research must revolve around understanding the factors that mediate the impact of chronic pruritus on QoL, with more frequent use of ItchyQoL, an itch-specific quality of life instrument [38]. A better appreciation of the complex relationship between chronic itch and quality of life can only improve the clinical evaluation and treatment of chronic pruritus [39]. Future directions along this line of research include investigating how race influences the impact of chronic pruritus on QoL, and exploring whether support groups or personality-specific interventions may help mitigate the QoL impact of chronic pruritus [39]. Finally, studies on itch threshold will enable a more accurate and objective measurement of pruritus.

From a basic science perspective, the renewed focus on itch as a specific target has led to the development of novel drugs that are currently being tested in clinically trials or that are currently under development. Among them are, for example, histamine H_4 receptor antagonists [40] and kappa-opioid receptor agonists that target the pruritic pathway directly [41, 42], and it is likely that additional drugs that target specific itch-related peptides or receptors will enter the clinic in the next decade. Cannabinoid receptor agonists have been demonstrated as effective topical modalities for itch treatment, although their potency in activating receptors can certainly be improved [33]. Further topical or systemic strategies using cannabinoid receptors as targets are promising for itch therapy. Biotechnological advances, for example the ability to generate humanized molecules targeting specific cellular structures, have made it possible to develop novel agents ("biologicals") such as the IL-4 and IL-4 receptor antagonists [43]. Other molecules, such as an anti-IL-31 receptor antibody [44], are being developed. In addition, novel oral treatments, such as the NK1 receptor-antagonist aprepitant, have just now been reported to be effective in various subforms of itch [45, 46].

Moving forward, targets on the therapeutic horizon are likely to include gastrin-releasing peptide and its receptor, which act on the level of the spinal cord and integrate many histamine- and histamine-independent itch pathways, as well as the protease pathway via activation of G protein-coupled protease-activated receptors [33].

Conclusion

Pruritus in old age is a debilitating and difficult symptom to treat, and has an overwhelmingly negative impact on the quality of life of those affected individuals. Decline in normal physiology of the skin, age-related changes in the immune system, polypharmacy, and other medical comorbidities all contribute to the high rate of pruritus in the elderly. These factors also make the diagnosis and its management more challenging. Fortunately, focusing on the basic principles of skin care can lead to safe and effective treatment of itch in the majority of elderly patients [2, 21, 30]. Treatment directed at the primary element triggering the pruritus is most effective. At times the pruritic elderly patient will have skin lesions induced by more than one of the age related processes, and treatment for each pathogenic process may be required [2]. The field eagerly awaits

38 K.C. Wang

future research to elucidate the pathological mechanisms underlying the myriad forms of pruritus, in order to bring therapeutic advances to the bedside.

References

1. Ständer S, Weisshaar E, Mettang T, et al. Clinical classification of itch: a position paper of the International Forum for the Study of Itch. Acta Derm Venereol. 2007;87:291–4.
2. Berger TG, Steinhoff M. Pruritus in elderly patients—eruptions of senescence. Semin Cutan Med Surg. 2011;30:113–7.
3. Bianchi J, Cameron J. Assessment of skin integrity in the elderly 1. Br J Community Nurs. 2008;13:S26–32.
4. Thaipisuttikul Y. Pruritic skin diseases in the elderly. J Dermatol. 1998;25:153–7.
5. Yalcin B, Tamer E, Toy GG, Oztaş P, Hayran M, Alli N. The prevalence of skin diseases in the elderly: analysis of 4099 geriatric patients. Int J Dermatol. 2006;45:672–6.
6. Beauregard S, Gilchrest BA. A survey of skin problems and skin care regimens in the elderly. Arch Dermatol. 1987;123:1638–43.
7. Norman RA, Henderson JN. Aging: an overview. Dermatol Ther. 2003;16:181–5.
8. Patel T, Yosipovitch G. Therapy of pruritus. Expert Opin Pharmacother. 2010;11:1673–82.
9. Shive M, Linos E, Berger T, Wehner M, Chren M-M. Itch as a patient-reported symptom in ambulatory care visits in the United States. J Am Acad Dermatol. 2013;69:550–6.
10. Fleischer Jr AB. Pruritus in the elderly: management by senior dermatologists. J Am Acad Dermatol. 1993;28:603–9.
11. Bernhard JD. Phantom itch, pseudophantom itch, and senile pruritus. Int J Dermatol. 1992;31:856–7.
12. Ward JR, Bernhard JD. Willan's itch and other causes of pruritus in the elderly. Int J Dermatol. 2005;44:267–73.
13. Norman RA. Geriatric dermatology. New York: Parthenon Publishing Group; 2001.
14. Weisshaar E, Dalgard F. Epidemiology of itch: adding to the burden of skin morbidity. Acta Derm Venereol. 2009;89:339–50.
15. Reich A, Ständer S, Szepietowski JC. Drug-induced pruritus: a review. Acta Derm Venereol. 2009;89:236–44.
16. Yosipovitch G, Bernhard JD. Clinical practice. Chronic pruritus. N Engl J Med. 2013;368:1625–34.
17. Kini SP, DeLong LK, Veledar E, McKenzie-Brown AM, Schaufele M, Chen SC. The impact of pruritus on quality of life: the skin equivalent of pain. Arch Dermatol. 2011;147:1153–6.
18. Reich A, Ständer S, Szepietowski JC. Pruritus in the elderly. Clin Dermatol. 2011;29:15–23.
19. Bigby M, Jick S, Jick H, Arndt K. Drug-induced cutaneous reactions. A report from the Boston Collaborative Drug Surveillance Program on 15,438 consecutive inpatients, 1975 to 1982. JAMA. 1986;256:3358–63.
20. Joly P, Benoit-Corven C, Baricault S, et al. Chronic eczematous eruptions of the elderly are associated with chronic exposure to calcium channel blockers: results from a case–control study. J Invest Dermatol. 2007;127:2766–71.
21. Berger TG, Shive M, Harper GM. Pruritus in the older patient: a clinical review. JAMA. 2013;310:2443–50.
22. Pawelec G, Larbi A, Derhovanessian E. Senescence of the human immune system. J Comp Pathol. 2010;142 Suppl 1:S39–44.
23. Weiskopf D, Weinberger B, Grubeck-Loebenstein B. The aging of the immune system. Transpl Int. 2009;22:1041–50.
24. Sandmand M, Bruunsgaard H, Kemp K, et al. Is ageing associated with a shift in the balance between Type 1 and Type 2 cytokines in humans? Clin Exp Immunol. 2002;127:107–14.
25. White-Chu EF, Reddy M. Dry skin in the elderly: complexities of a common problem. Clin Dermatol. 2011;29:37–42.
26. Veien NKN, Laurberg GG. Brachioradial pruritus: a follow-up of 76 patients. Acta Derm Venereol. 2011;91:183–5.
27. Yilmaz S, Ceyhan AM, Akkaya VB. Brachioradial pruritus successfully treated with gabapentin. J Dermatol. 2010;37:662–5.
28. De Ridder D, Hans G, Pals P, Menovsky T. A C-fiber-mediated neuropathic brachioradial pruritus. J Neurosurg. 2010;113(1):118–21. http://dx.doi.org/10.3171/2009.9.JNS09620.
29. Yamaoka H, Sasaki H, Yamasaki H, et al. Truncal pruritus of unknown origin may be a symptom of diabetic polyneuropathy. Diabetes Care. 2010;33:150–5.
30. Garibyan L, Chiou AS, Elmariah SB. Advanced aging skin and itch: addressing an unmet need. Dermatol Ther. 2013;26:92–103.
31. Dupont C, de Maubeuge J, Kotlar W, Lays Y, Masson M. Oxatomide in the treatment of pruritus senilis. Dermatology. 1984;169:348–53.
32. American Geriatrics Society 2012 Beers Criteria Update Expert Panel. American Geriatrics Society updated Beers Criteria for potentially inappropriate medication use in older adults. J Am Geriatr Soc. 2012;60:616–31.
33. Steinhoff MM, Cevikbas FF, Ikoma AA, Berger TGT. Pruritus: management algorithms and experimental therapies. Semin Cutan Med Surg. 2011;30:127–37.
34. Rivard J, Lim HW. Ultraviolet phototherapy for pruritus. Dermatol Ther. 2005;18:344–54.
35. Seckin D, Demircay Z, Akin O. Generalized pruritus treated with narrowband UVB. Int J Dermatol. 2007;46:367–70.

36. Rombold S, Lobisch K, Katzer K, Grazziotin TC, Ring J, Eberlein B. Efficacy of UVA1 phototherapy in 230 patients with various skin diseases. Photodermatol Photoimmunol Photomed. 2008;24:19–23.
37. Pisoni RLR, Wikström B, Elder SJ, et al. Pruritus in haemodialysis patients: international results from the Dialysis Outcomes and Practice Patterns Study (DOPPS). Nephrol Dial Transplant. 2006;21:3495–505.
38. Desai NS, Poindexter GB, Monthrope YM, Bendeck SE, Swerlick RA, Chen SC. A pilot quality-of-life instrument for pruritus. J Am Acad Dermatol. 2008;59:234–44.
39. Carr CW, Veledar E, Chen SC. Factors mediating the impact of chronic pruritus on quality of life. JAMA Dermatol. 2014;150:613–20.
40. Dunford PJ, Williams KN, Desai PJ, Karlsson L, McQueen D, Thurmond RL. Histamine H4 receptor antagonists are superior to traditional antihistamines in the attenuation of experimental pruritus. J Allergy Clin Immunol. 2007;119:176–83.
41. Kumagai H, Ebata T, Takamori K, Muramatsu T, Nakamoto H, Suzuki H. Effect of a novel kappa-receptor agonist, nalfurafine hydrochloride, on severe itch in 337 haemodialysis patients: a phase III, randomized, double-blind, placebo-controlled study. Nephrol Dial Transplant. 2010;25:1251–7.
42. Phan NQ, Lotts T, Antal A, Bernhard JD, Ständer S. Systemic kappa opioid receptor agonists in the treatment of chronic pruritus: a literature review. Acta Derm Venereol. 2012;92:555–60.
43. Beck LA, Thaçi D, Hamilton JD, et al. Dupilumab treatment in adults with moderate-to-severe atopic dermatitis. N Engl J Med. 2014;371:130–9.
44. Kasutani K, Fujii E, Ohyama S, et al. Anti-IL-31 receptor antibody is shown to be a potential therapeutic option for treating itch and dermatitis in mice. Br J Pharmacol. 2014. doi:10.1111/bph.12823.
45. Santini D, Vincenzi B, Guida FM, et al. Aprepitant for management of severe pruritus related to biological cancer treatments: a pilot study. Lancet Oncol. 2012;13:1020–4.
46. Torres TT, Fernandes II, Selores MM, Alves RR, Lima MM. Aprepitant: evidence of its effectiveness in patients with refractory pruritus continues. J Am Acad Dermatol. 2012;66:e14–5.

Aged-Related Changes in the Nails

John Montgomery Yost

Introduction

Nail changes and disorders are common among elderly individuals, and occur at different rates when compared to the general population. The nail apparatus ages intrinsically, resulting in certain characteristic clinical changes [1]. Conversely, nail disorders are acquired and arise from secondary pathologic processes. It is important for clinicians to be familiar with both categories and differentiate between the two.

Nail Changes in Older Adults

Classically, the clinical manifestations of the aging nail have been defined as changes in nail plate color, contour, linear growth, surface, and thickness [2]. These alterations likely result from a multifactorial process, including arteriosclerosis or impaired peripheral circulation, ultraviolet radiation, trauma, and faulty biomechanics [3].

In the normal nail, the color of nail plate is white immediately above the lunula, the visible and most distal aspect of the nail matrix, and pink in the portion overlying the nail bed [4]. In contrast, the nails of the elderly are often yellow, grey or white [4]. Such whitening of the nail plate overlying the nail bed is termed leukonychia, and may result from age-related changes of the nail matrix resulting in opacity of the nail plate (true leukonychia) or the nail bed (apparent leukonychia). With age, the lunula also significantly decreases in size, and may completely vanish [3–5]. Other specific well-described variations in nail plate color—including Terry's nails, half-and-half nails, and Muehrcke's lines—also occur in elderly individuals, though they are often associated with underlying systemic diseases [6–8].

Contour related nail changes vary between fingernails and toenails. With age, the longitudinal curvature of fingernails often deceases, resulting in a flat (platyonychia) or concave (koilonychias) nail plate [3, 4]. The latter condition is notably associated with many other congenital and acquired pathologic processes and thus is not specific for aging [9]. Nail clubbing also occurs in elderly individuals, however, is associated with underlying bronchopulmonary disease in the majority of all cases [9].

Increased transverse curvature of the nail plate represents the most common age-related change in toenails. Radiographic data confirm that this change directly results from progressive widening of the base of the distal phalanx and thus affecting the overlying nail matrix [10]. Consequently, as the proximal nail plate progressively flattens, the transverse curvature of

J.M. Yost, M.D., M.P.H. (✉)
Assistant Professor, Department of Dermatology,
Stanford University School of Medicine,
450 Broadway Street, Pavilion C,
Redwood City, CA 94063, USA
e-mail: johnmyost@gmail.com

© Springer International Publishing Switzerland 2015
A.L.S. Chang (ed.), *Advances in Geriatric Dermatology*, DOI 10.1007/978-3-319-18380-0_3

the distal plate increases to compensate in a lever-like manner [10]. Such changes often result in the painful incarceration of the distal nail bed between the lateral aspects of the nail plate, a condition termed "pincer nail deformity" or onychocryptosis [10]. In addition to intrinsic aging, acquired pincer nail deformity is also clinically associated with various tumors of the nail apparatus, systemic medications (with β-blockers being the most common), underlying visceral and hematologic malignancies, end stage renal failure, and autoimmune disease [10–14]. Given the intrinsic distal nature of the location, conservative interventions are often favored initially for this condition, including mechanical thinning of the nail plate, chemical softening of the nail plate with keratolytics or acids, and trimming of the lateral aspects of the nail [10, 15]. Mechanical bracing of the affected nails using a technique termed orthonyx has also been attempted with encouraging results [16, 17]. Specifically, a memory alloy prosthesis is attached to the lateral aspects of the nail in order to exert pressure opposing the transverse nail curvature, thus flattening the plate [16, 17]. Surgical intervention is often required in cases recalcitrant to conservative therapies, with cauterization of the lateral matrical horns and dermal grafting under the nail matrix providing the most consistent, permanent results [10, 18, 19].

The rate of linear nail growth has been well demonstrated to progressively decrease with advanced age. The physiologic average rate of linear growth is 0.1 mm/day (3.0 mm/month) for fingernails and 0.03 mm/day (1.0 mm/month) for toenails until the age of 25, at which time this rate decreases approximately by 0.5 %/year [20]. Concomitant systemic disease and medications may also alter linear nail growth [3].

Onychorrhexis, or the superficial longitudinal ridging of the dorsal nail plate, represents the most characteristic age-related change in nail plate surface, and likely results from a disregulation in nail matrix keratinocyte turnover [21]. In some cases these ridges may also act as a nidus for plate to split distally, most often distal to the hyponychium. As such, affected individuals are frequently distressed by the cosmesis of these changes, even though there is no associated medical risk or functional impairment. Periodic nail plate buffing is considered the most effective therapeutic intervention, though caution is recommended in patients with preexisting age-related nail plate thinning or atrophy, as any mechanical manipulation may paradoxically increase the risk of nail plate splitting [4].

Nail plate thickness represents the distance between dorsal and ventral surfaces, and is determined by the length of the nail matrix. However, both environmental and systemic factors may also contribute to nail plate hypertrophy or atrophy. In general, toenails often thicken with age, while fingernails often become thinner [22]. Such changes may affect one or all of nails [22]. Specifically, the idiopathic thickening of an isolated nail plate is termed onychauxis, while thickening of all ten toenails is referred to as pachyonychia. In extreme cases, the nail plate may develop an ostraceous or "ram's horn-like appearance" (given the nail curvature and hypertrophy), termed onychogryphosis (Fig. 1). While these changes can occur on any of the digits, the hallux is most commonly affected. Treatment for nail plate hypertrophy is generally recommended to prevent self-injury and unintended excoriations, and typically entails either chemical or mechanical debridement [4]. Notably, mechanical debridement is often most successful when performed by a provider, as some elderly individuals may experience difficulty with the posturing and dexterity necessary. Complete avulsion of the nail plate without matrix ablation is a therapeutic alternative in refractory cases [4].

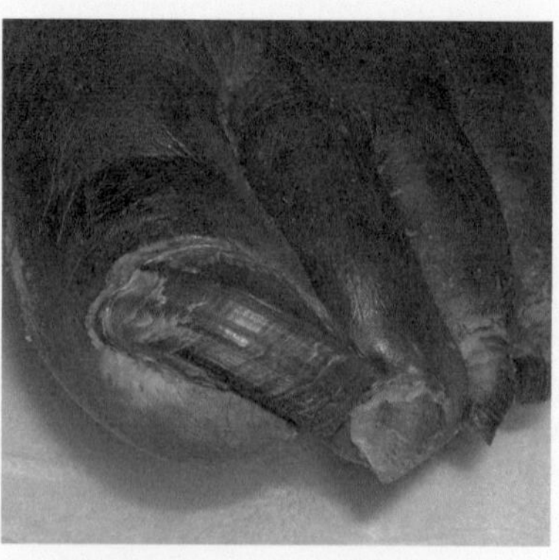

Fig. 1 Onychogryphosis

Common Nail Disorders in Older Adults

In addition to the intrinsic physiologic changes of the nail plate that occur with aging, nail disorders are common in geriatric populations. This high prevalence of nail disease in the elderly is multi-factorial: impaired circulation, increased suscep-tibility of the nail apparatus to infection due to barrier defects, increased rate of cutaneous neo-plasms, elevated prevalence of comorbid derma-tologic or systemic disease, and medication use are all contributing factors [2].

Brittle Nail Disease

While largely a cosmetic concern, nail brittleness is a common complaint of elderly individuals, occurring in an estimated 35 % of individuals older than 60 years [23]. Typically, affected indi-viduals complain of soft, easily torn or split nails, and a general inability to grow longer nails [4]. As described above, longitudinal nail splitting occurs commonly in the setting of intrinsic age-related onychorrhexis (Fig. 2). Onychoschizia—or the distal lamellar peeling and splitting of the dorsal aspect of the nail plate—also is common in the elderly, particularly women, as is trachyonychia—an opaque roughness affecting the surface of the dorsal nail plate.

Previously, brittle nails were believed to result from decreased water content. However, this theory has since been disproved, with emerging data now demonstrating no significant difference in water content between normal and brittle nails [24]. Instead, water binding capac-ity has been identified as the likely causative factor, as it is reduced by nearly one half in brittle nail plates [25, 26]. As keratin, keratin-associated proteins, and lipid-content all con-tribute to nail plate water binding capacity, an abnormality in one or several of these factors may underlie brittle nail pathophysiology [27, 28]. Environmental factors may also further exacer-bate brittle nails clinically, though they are not believed to represent a causative factor [29]. Patients with brittle nails are advised to avoid repeated hydration and desiccation of the nail plates (which often occurs occupational set-tings) as well as exposure to dehydrating agents used in nail cosmetics, as these may damage intracellular corneocyte bridges and dissolving intracellular lipids, thereby further increasing nail plate fragility [29, 30]. Rarely, brittle nails may also represent a harbinger of an underlying dermatologic or systemic disease, including psoriasis, lichen planus, lichen striatus, alopecia areata, Darier's disease, peripheral arterial disease, arteriosclerosis, microangiopathy, Raynaud's disease, polycythemia vera, dyserythropoietic anemia, thyroid disease, hypopituitarism, gout,

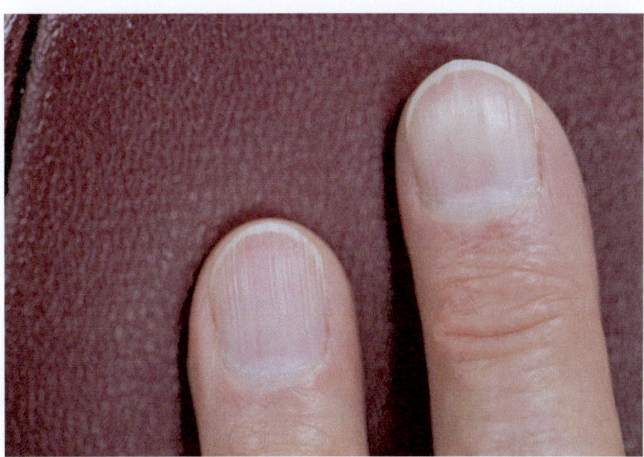

Fig. 2 Onychorrhexis

osteoporosis, diabetes, malnutrition and nutritional disorders, chronic renal failure, hemodialysis, osteomalacia, acromegaly, pulmonary tuberculosis, chronic obstructive pulmonary disease, sarcoidosis, systemic amyloidosis, and various visceral malignancies—often in the setting of acrokeratosis paraneoplastica [31–36].

Treatment of brittle nails is often difficult given the multifactorial nature of the disease. As stated previously, environmental exposures may exacerbate any underlying nail disease, and patients should be advised to reduce frequency of prolonged contact with water, as well as detergents, cleaning solvents, and alcohol-based hand sanitizers [30]. For prolonged contact with water, cotton-lined latex gloves should be worn. Hydration of the nail plate is also essential and patients should be advised to apply a thick emollient to the entire nail plate and proximal nail fold after soaking the tips in lukewarm water for 10–20 min [37]. Urea and lactic acid have been reported as particularly effective, as both agents act to increase the water content binding capacity of the nail plate [30]. Nail cosmetics may be cautiously recommended, as once-weekly application of nail lacquer may limit exposure of water and other offending detergents, as well as reduce water vapor loss [38]. However, since acetone, and to a lesser degree acetate, dehydrate the nail plate and reduce the intrinsic lipid content, polish removers should be used on a very limited basis [38]. Cosmetic nail hardeners should also be recommended judiciously, as they contain toluene-sulfonamide-formaldehyde resins, which induce additional cross-linking between nail plate keratin. While such bonds may help to stabilize weakened nails, overuse may result in accumulation of excess keratin cross-links, thus paradoxically decreasing nail plate flexibility and increasing brittleness [38].

More recently, two new prescription medications targeting brittle nails have been released. The first agent recently gained FDA approval as a medical device for the treatment of brittle nails, and consists of a hydrosoluble nail lacquer containing hydroxypropyl chitosan, *Equisetum avense* extract and methylsulfonyl methane, which is marketed under the trade name *Genadur*®

(distributed by Medimetriks). In one study, daily applications of this agent significantly reduced longitudinal groves and lamellar splitting after 1 month [39]. The second agent, a 16 % urea polyurethane lacquer, marketed as *Nu-Vail*® (distributed by Innocutis) also recently gained FDA approval as a medical device for the treatment of dystrophic nails, and was found to demonstrate a 60 % improvement in clinical parameters after 6 months of daily use [40]. Biotin supplementation can also often recommended as a systemic agent for the treatment of brittle nails, as elevated doses have been suggested to upregulate the synthesis of lipid molecules in the nail matrix, thus facilitating binding between nail plate keratinocytes [41]. Typically, dosages of 2.5–5 mg/day are recommended, as one study demonstrated a 25 % increase in nail thickness and an overall decrease in lamellar splitting with this agent [41]. Tazarotene 0.1 % cream has also anecdotally been suggested as a possible therapy, though few data exist [42].

Onychomycosis and Its Treatment in Older Adults

Onychomycosis is defined as a fungal infection that affects one or more components of the nail apparatus, with dermatophytes, yeasts, and non-dermatophytes molds all recognized as causative pathogens [43]. While the prevalence of such infections is approximately 10 % in the general population, upwards of 40–60 % of individuals over 60 years of age are affected [44, 45]. This overrepresentation of onychomycosis in geriatric populations is likely multifactorial, with reduced peripheral circulation, slower nail plate growth, inactivity, relative immunosuppression, glucose intolerance, larger distorted nail surfaces, difficulty with routine nail care and hygiene, increased risk of nail injury, and increased exposure to pathogenic fungi all representing contributing etiologic factors [3, 46].

Onychomycosis has a number of well-described common clinical presentations [47]. Of these, distolateral subungual onychomycosis is by far the most common, and is frequently associated with *Trichophyton* spp. (particularly *T. rubrum* and *T. mentagrophytes*). In this entity, the point of fungal entry is either the hyponychium or the lateral nail bed, resulting in the classic clinical presentation of distal onycholysis, subungual hyperkeratosis with an accumulation of subungal debris, and a thickened nail plate. Conversely, proximal subungual onychomycosis is the rarest clinical variant, and is most often associated with underlying human immunodeficiency virus infection [48]. *Trichophyton rubrum* is the most common causative organism associated with this condition [49]. As the infection originates at the proximal nail fold and spreads distally, clinically presenting as an opaque white discoloration of the proximal nail plate immediately overlying the lunula [43]. White superficial onychomycosis, a third clinical variant, involves the dorsal surface of the nail plate, and presents with coalescing opaque patches. The most common associated pathogen, *Trichophyton mentagrophytes*, contains enzymes capable of degrading nail plate keratins, so that affected areas appear crumbled and dilapidated [43].

Though many clinicians initiate treatment of onychomycosis based on clinical impression alone, this is not recommended as many other entities present with similar clinical findings. Pathologic diagnosis can easily be obtained through periodic-acid Schiff (PAS) staining of nail clippings or subungual debris, though it cannot reliably speciate the infecting organisms. Additionally, the pathologic diagnosis relies on the presence of branching septae; yeast forms alone do not confirm fungal infection of the nail apparatus [50]. Culture remains the gold standard for diagnosis, as it also identifies the pathogenic organism and allows antifungal sensitivity testing, though has a relatively low sensitivity of 53 % [51]. Accordingly, best practice guidelines dictate that both culture and PAS staining should be performed, as this combination yields a sensitivity of 96 % [51].

Treatment of onychomycosis in elderly populations has traditionally been difficult, primarily due to poor response, frequent relapses, and elevated associated risk profiles [3]. Topical therapy definitively carries the lowest risk of toxicity, though has historically not been curative. Instead, topical treatments have often been employed as a palliative measures, preventing the spread of fungal infection to neighboring nails. Ciclopirox 8 % lacquer is the most well studied topical agent, demonstrating clinical cure in 5.5–8.5 % of all cases [52]. Urea 40 % gel has also been anecdotally recommended as an adjunctive agent, theoretically increasing cutaneous absorption of any topical antifungal preparation [53]. However, the recent FDA approval of two new topical agents for will likely affect the treatment algorithm for onychomycosis, particularly in elderly adults.

Efinaconazole (Jublia® distributed by Valeant) is a new triazole antifungal topical solution that received FDA approval in June 2014 for the treatment of onychomycosis. Data from duplicate industry-sponsored phase III clinical studies demonstrated that 17.8 and 15.2 % of all study subjects attained a complete cure after 52 weeks of daily treatment [54]. An additional 35.7 and 31.0 % of study subjects were also noted to have less than 10 % of nail plate involvement after completing the treatment regimen. The most common attributable adverse reactions reported during the preclinical studies were application site dermatitis (3.5 %), application site vesicles (2.0 %, 1.2 %), contact dermatitis (2.9 %, 1.4 %) and ingrowing nail (2.6 %, 1.9 %), though one subsequent smaller study suggests the ability of efinaconazole to induce delayed contact sensitivity may be limited [54, 55].

Tavaborole (Kerydin® distributed by Anacor Pharmaceuticals), a first-in-class, boron-containing oxaborole broad-spectrum with antifungal activity against dermatophytes, yeast, and non-dermatophyte molds, also recently received FDA approval for the treatment of onychomycosis [56]. In duplicate industry-sponsored phase III clinical trials, complete clinical cure was achieved 6.5 and 9.1 % of patients treated with tavaborole for 360 days [57]. An "almost clear nail" was also observed in an additional 26.1 and 27.5 % of study subjects. In both the phase II and phase III clinical trials, adverse events were infrequent and limited to cutaneous irritation [57].

Regardless of the topical agent selected, the infected portion of the nail plate should be frequently debrided, ideally every 3–4 weeks [4]. Removal of the affected nail plate and subungual debris not only decreases fungal load, but also may increase topical therapy penetration [58]. While topical therapies carry a very low risk of toxicity, compliance with daily or twice daily applications can be difficulty for elderly individuals, particularly in the setting of limited mobility or other musculoskeletal or rheumatologic comorbidities [59].

Surgical or chemical nail avulsion represents an additional adjunctive therapy that best utilized in cases with lateral nail plate involvement [60]. The presence of a dermatophytoma—a subungual mass of densely packed fungal hyphae with poor antifungal penetration—is another indication for partial or complete nail debridement [60, 61].

Systemic antifungal therapy remains the gold standard for treatment of onychomycosis. Terbinafine, fluconazole, and itraconazole are the three agents most widely prescribed systemic antifungals. Due to the safety and efficacy concerns, older agents such as griseofulvin and ketoconazole are infrequently prescribed. Of the former three, only terbinafine and itraconazole are FDA-approved for the treatment of onychomycosis. Prior to the initiation of any systemic treatment regimen, the following factors should be considered: the patient's relevant past medical history, current medications, and the causative or suspected pathogen.

Terbinafine is a synthetic allylamine antifungal with fungicidal activity against fungi, dermatophytes, and some yeast forms through the inhibition of squalene epoxidase [62]. This agent is currently the drug of choice for treating onychomycosis, as it has been repeatedly demonstrated to have the highest rates of clinical cure and the lowest rates of recurrence [63–65]. Terbinafine is also highly lipophilic and persists in the nail plate for several months after discontinuation [62]. Terbinafine is dosed at 250 mg daily for 6 weeks for fingernail onychomycosis and 12 weeks for toenail onychomycosis. The data regarding the overall efficacy rate for terbinafine

vary. Several meta-analyses suggest a clinical cure rate between 66 and 75 %, though early studies demonstrate rates of 38–54 % [65–69]. Adverse effects commonly attributed to terbinafine include nausea, gastrointestinal disturbance, dysgeusia, leukopenia, liver function abnormalities, and cutaneous eruption [43]. Rarely, terbinafine has been associated with fulminant liver failure, and thus, intermittent laboratory assessment of hepatic parameters is often performed. Terbinafine has few significant drug interactions, and can be co-administered statins, digoxin, warfarin, and many other medications commonly prescribed in elderly populations [43]. However, this agent is a potent inhibitor of CYP2D6, affecting the metabolism of numerous medications including many beta-blockers as well as donepezil, and thus, medication reconciliation and review is recommended prior to initiating therapy [70]. In older patients who may be on multiple medications (including hepatically metabolized drugs such as statins), pulse dose treatment consisting of 7 days a month for 4 months has been shown to reduce likelihood of transaminitis with only slightly lower cure rates [67].

Itraconazole is a synthetic triazole antifungal, and has a broad spectrum of fungistatic activity but potential side effects with older adults should be carefully considered [71]. Through the inhibition of ergosterol synthesis, itraconazole is able to inhibit growth of dermatophytes, *Candida*, and some nondermatophyte molds [71]. Similar to terbinafine, itraconazole is also highly lipophilic and persists in the nail plate for 6–9 months after discontinuation [71]. Two dosing regimens exist for itraconazole: daily treatment and intermittent (pulse) therapy. Daily treatment is dosed at 200 mg/day for 8 weeks for fingernail onychomycosis and 12 weeks for toenail onychomycosis. Pulse therapy, which is not FDA-approved for the treatment of toenail onychomycosis, consists of 400 mg/day for the first week of every month and lasts 2 months for fingernail onychomycosis and 3 months for toenail onychomycosis. As with terbinafine, the data regarding the efficacy of itraconazole vary, though most larger and head-to-head studies suggest terbinafine has a higher overall clinical cure rate than either of the itraconazole dosing regimens [65, 66, 68]. Notably, itraconazole is absolutely contraindicated in patients with a past medical history of congestive heart failure due to its negative inotropic effect [72]. Other associated adverse reactions include nausea, gastrointestinal disturbance, telogen effluvium, hepatotoxicity, and cutaneous eruption [43]. Itraconazole is also a potent inhibitor of CYP3A4, and thus interacts with many medications. Those specifically mentioned in the associated FDA-mandated black box warning include: cisapride, midazolam, nisoldipine, felodipine, pimozide, quinidine, dofetilide, triazolam, levacetylmethadol, lovastatin, simvastatin, ergot alkaloids, and methadone [73]. Given these associations and interactions, itraconazole is not typically a first-line agent in onychomycosis among elderly populations, though it has a definite clinical value in certain settings [74].

Of note, two published, peer-reviewed studies exist that specifically pertain to the treatment of onychomycosis in the elderly. The first—a single blind, randomized, non-industry-sponsored, prospective study—compared the efficacy of terbinafine and itraconazole in the treatment of onychomycosis [75]. In total, 101 individuals aged 60 years and older with dermatophytosis involving at least one hallux were enrolled. Half were treated with terbinafine 250 mg daily for 12 weeks, while the remaining individuals were treated with itraconazole 200 mg twice daily for 1 week per month for 3 months [75]. The resulting data demonstrated no significant difference in cure rates: the clinical cure rates were 62 % for terbinafine and 60.8 % for itraconazole [75]. Adverse events were noted in five individuals in the terbinafine treatment group and seven individuals in the itraconazole treatment group, all of which were mild and reversible [75]. The second study performed a subanalysis of patients 65 years and older from an open-label, randomized, multicenter study of adults treated with terbinafine or terbinafine and surgical nail debridement for onychomycosis [76]. Specifically, surgical nail debridement in the context of onychomycosis traditionally refers to the removal of all onycholytic portions of the nail plate, thus reducing the fungal load by eliminating the subungual debris [76]. The resulting data demonstrated that patients treated with both terbinafine and surgical debridement had higher rates of complete cure than those treated with terbinafine alone [76]. Additionally, the most frequently reported adverse events included nausea, arthralgia, and hypercholesterolemia, with three participants ultimately withdrawing due to a medication-related adverse effect [76]. Of the enrolled individuals 97 % of patients were concomitantly taking another oral medication throughout the course of the study: 64 % antihypertensives, 25 % antidiabetics, and 47 % lipid-lowering medications [76].

Lastly, various lasers and other light-based devices have been posited as a potential alternative therapeutic modality for onychomycosis, although their exact mechanism of action is unclear. Currently, the five devices are currently approved by the FDA for the treatment of onychomycosis, all of which are short-pulse neodymium-doped yttrium aluminum garnet (Nd:Yag) lasers [77]. Notably, all five devices only received approval for temporary increase in clear nail in patients with onychomycosis, not definitive treatment [78]. While the idea of laser treatment for onycomycosis seems promising, to date the data supporting the actual efficacy of this modality is mixed. One review of all relevant published studies pertaining to treatment of onychomycosis with the Nd:Yag reemphasized that while results were favorable, all studies were small and many poorly designed [77]. Furthermore, a more recent larger, randomized controlled trial found no significant difference in mycological culture or nail plate clearance [78].

Nail-Associated Neoplasms in the Elderly

Tumors of the nail unit can be classified as benign, malignant, or metastatic. While fibrous tumors are the most common neoplasms of the nail apparatus in the general population, digital myxoid cysts predominate as the most prevalent among the elderly [3, 79, 80]. These tumors have

Fig. 3 Glomus tumor

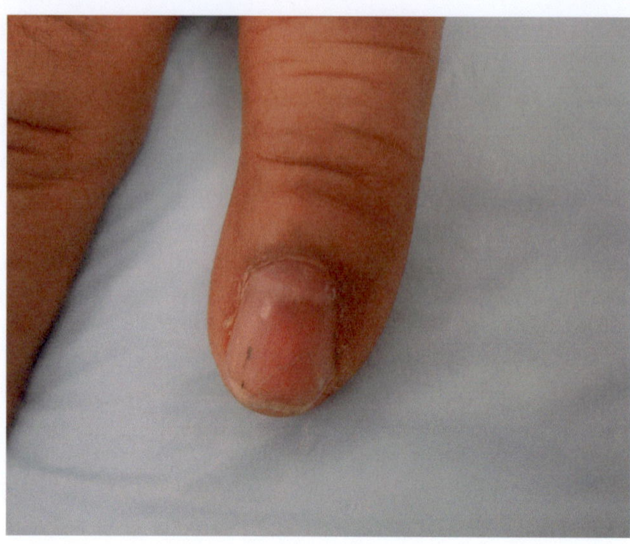

many synonyms, including pseudomyxoid cysts, ganglion cysts, and digital mucous cysts, focal mucinosis, periarticular fibromas, and cutaneous myxoid cysts, among others [81, 82]. Digital myxoid cysts classically present as skin-colored to blue, smooth, translucent, dome-shaped papule located distal to the distal interphalangeal (DIP) joint, most commonly on the first three fingers [3, 81]. Histopathologically, these lesions are characterized by a deep focal mucinosis on acral skin without an epithelial lining. In over 80 % of cases digital myxoid cysts connect with the underlying DIP joint [83]. In cases where the lesion is located more distally and involves the proximal nail fold, the lesion may compress the underlying nail matrix and result in a longitudinal grove in the nail plate [81]. Generally, asymptomatic digital myxoid cysts are best observed clinically. For symptomatic or cosmetically bothersome lesions, surgical excision with ligation of communicating tract to the underlying joint is the gold standard for treatment [84]. Simple drainage of the lesions is a less invasive alternative for patients unwilling or unable to undergo surgery, though it is also associated with higher rates of recurrence [85].

Glomus tumors represent another common benign neoplasm involving the nail unit. While glomus tumors can develop at any site on the body, upwards of 75 % occur on the hand, most commonly on the fingertips [81]. Epidemiologically, over 90 % of cases occur in women, with an average age of 45 years [86]. Glomus tumors have two distinct clinical presentations: (1) a small red or blue macule on the nail bed that is visible through the nail plate (Fig. 3), or (2) longitudinal erythronychia—or a longitudinal erythematous streak that extends the length of the nail bed visible through the nail plate— with an overlying furrow in the nail plate and distal nicking [87]. The characteristic triad of associated pain, pinpoint tenderness and temperature (especially cold) sensitivity is highly specific in reaching a diagnosis [87]. Magnetic resonance imaging can be used to confirm the diagnosis in most cases. This imaging modality has the best capacity to assess the size and extent of the lesion and provides the highest sensitivity amongst all imaging modalities [88–90]. Surgical excision the primary treatment for these tumors, though some evidence suggests a recurrence rate of approximately 17 % [91]. Asymptomatic lesions can be monitored clinically, though further evaluation and biopsy are recommended if squamous cell carcinoma or amelanotic melanoma is in the differential diagnosis.

Squamous cell carcinoma is the most common malignant neoplasm affecting the nail apparatus [81, 87]. While epidemiologic data for this malignancy is limited, one retrospective study found a male predominance, with a peak incidence between 50 and 69 years of age [92]. Risk factors for subungual or periungual squamous cell carcinoma include: trauma, ionizing radiation, arsenic exposure, dyskeratosis congenita, and human papillomavirus (HPV) infection [92–94]. Specifically, HPV subtype 16 DNA has been identified by polymerase chain reaction (PCR) in 74 % of all reported cases [93]. The morphologic presentation of squamous cell carcinoma of the nail unit can be variable and may mimic a variety of benign conditions clinically, often delaying diagnosis and appropriate treatment [87, 95]. While subungual involvement is most common, tumors may also arise in the paronychial epithelium [87]. Subungual lesions typically present with onycholysis overlying a verrucous or hyperkeratotic mass or a frank ulcer (Fig. 4) [87]. The loss of any longitudinal portion of nail plate indicates involvement of the matrix. Periungual lesions classically present as painless, slow-growing, hyperkeratotic or verrucous, papules or tumors that may ulcerate or bleed [81]. Mohs micrographic surgery is the treatment of choice for all squamous cell carcinomas involving the nail unit as it has the highest cure rate [96]. Nonetheless, recurrences still occur in as many as 20 % of cases [93]. Long standing lesions may progress to involve bone in between 20 and 60 % of patients [81, 97]. In cases of bone invasion, amputation of the distal phalanx is recommended by most sources [95].

Melanoma of the nail apparatus is a relatively rare malignancy in individuals of Caucasian descent, accounting for 1.4–3 % of all melanomas in this group [99–101]. Notably, while the relative incidence of nail unit melanoma is significantly higher among populations of color—with rates reported between 17 and 25 %—the absolute incidence does not differ significantly between ethnic groups [102–104]. Data from several large epidemiological studies suggests that the peak incidence occurs at approximately 60 years of age, with no significant difference between the sexes [99, 100, 105–108]. Most cases of nail unit melanoma

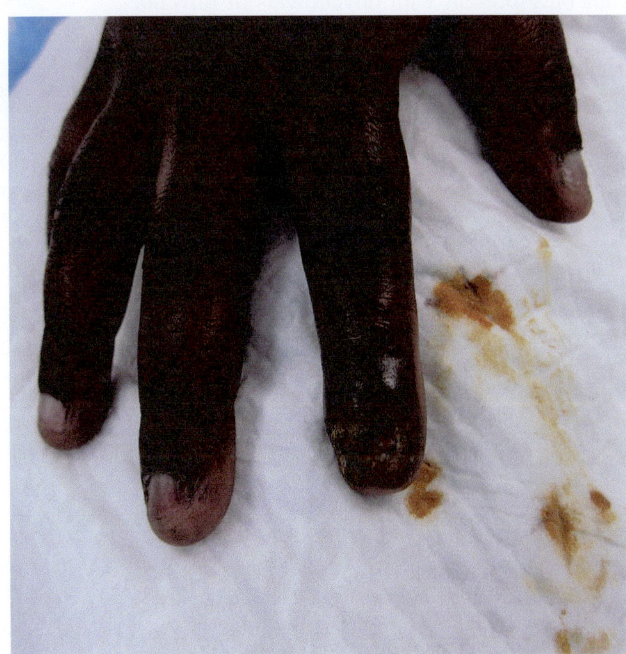

Fig. 4 Subungual squamous cell carcinoma

arise from the nail matrix, though tumors arising in the nail bed and lateral nail folds have also been reported [109]. The thumbs and halluces are most the most common sites, likely due to the increased proportion of nail matrix on digits, with no significant difference between left and right sides [103, 110]. The clinical presentation of nail unit melanoma largely is determined by the site of origin. Longitudinal melanonychia is the most common presenting sign and occurs in approximately 76 % of cases [111]. As longitudinal melanonychia may also result from benign lesions, the "ABCDEF rule" [Table 1] was developed to assist clinicians in identifying suspicious lesions requiring additional evaluation [112]. Hutchinson's sign—defined as pigment extension onto the proximal nail fold, lateral nail folds, or hyponychium—often represents the radial growth phase of melanoma arising in the nail matrix [113]. While Hutchinson's sign is by no mean pathognomonic for subungual melanoma, its presence almost always necessitates a biopsy. In addition to longitudinal melanonychia, other presenting signs include nail plate thinning and fissuring. It is important to note that upwards 20 % of nail unit melanomas are amelanotic, and thus only present with onycholysis or onychorrhexis affecting a solitary digit [114, 115]. Historically, amputation of the all or a portion of the affected digit was recommended for all cases of nail unit melanoma. However, these guidelines are now being reevaluated given the significant morbidity associated with the complete loss of a digit and the lack of evidence of a definitive survival benefit from amputation [116]. As such, some clinicians are performing wide local excisions such as degloving procedures for more superficial lesions [108].

Conclusions

Increased age confers increased risk of nail-associated malignancy and timely biopsy is essential to early detection. Older adults are also more likely to use multiple medications, which have the potential to interact with common treatments for onychomycosis, a widespread condition in this population. Recent studies in the elderly population have begun to explore safer and more effective ways to treat onychomycosis.

Table 1 ABCDEFs of nail melanoma

A	*Age*: peak incidence at 60 years of age *Race*: African-American, Asian, Native American
B	*Band Pigment*: Brown-Black *Breadth*: ≥3 mm *Border*: irregular, blurred
C	*Change*: rapid increase in size, growth of nail band *Lack of Change*: failure of dystrophy to improve despite adequate treatment
D	*Digit Involved*: Thumb, Hallux > index finger *Dominant Hand*
E	*Extension*: pigment extending to involve proximal/lateral nail fold, hyponychium, free nail plate edge
F	*Family or Personal History* of previous melanoma

Reprinted with permission from ref. [112]

References

1. Chang AL, Wong JW, Endo JO, Norman RA. Geriatric dermatology review: major changes in skin function in older patients and their contribution to common clinical challenges. J Am Med Dir Assoc. 2013;14(10):724–30.
2. Cohen PR, Scher RK. Geriatric nail disorders: diagnosis and treatment. J Am Acad Dermatol. 1992; 26(4):521–31.
3. de Berker DAR, Richert B, Baran R. The nail in childhood and old age. In: Baran R, de Berker DAR, Holzbert M, Thomas L, editors. Baran & Dawber's diseases of the nails and their management. 4th ed. Oxford: Blackwell; 2012. p. 183–209.
4. Cohen PR, Scher RK. Nails in older individuals. In: Scher RK, Daniel CR, editors. Nails: diagnosis, therapy, surgery. 3rd ed. Philadelphia: Saunders; 2005. p. 245–64.
5. Cohen PR. The lunula. J Am Acad Dermatol. 1996; 34(6):943–53.
6. Terry R. White nails in hepatic cirrhosis. Lancet. 1954;266(6815):757–9.
7. Lindsay PG. The half-and-half nail. Arch Intern Med. 1967;119(6):583–7.
8. Muehrcke RC. The finger-nails in chronic hypoalbuminaemia: a new physical sign. Br Med J. 1956; 1(4979):1327–8.
9. Stone OJ. Clubbing and koilonychia. Dermatol Clin. 1985;3(3):485–90.
10. Baran R, Haneke E, Richert B. Pincer nails: definition and surgical treatment. Dermatol Surg. 2001; 27(3):261–6.

11. Baran R, Broutard JC. Epidermoid cyst of the thumb presenting as pincer nail. J Am Acad Dermatol. 1998;19:143–4.

12. Greiner D, Schöfer H, Milbradt R. Reversible transverse overcurvature of the nails (pincer nails) after treatment with a β-blocker. J Am Acad Dermatol. 1998;39:486–7.

13. Jemec GBE, Thomsen K. Pincer nails and alopecia as markers of gastrointestinal malignancy. J Dermatol. 1997;24:479–81.

14. Majeski C, Richie B, Giuffre M, Lauzon G. Pincer nail deformity associated with systemic lupus erythematosis. J Cutan Med Surg. 2005;9(1):2–5.

15. Okada K, Okada E. Novel treatment using thioglycolic acid for pincer nails. J Dermatol. 2012;39(12): 996–9.

16. Tseng JT, Ho WT, Hsu CH, Lin MH, Li CN, Lee WR. A simple therapeutic approach to pincer nail deformity using a memory alloy: measurement of response. Dermatol Surg. 2013;39(3):398–405.

17. Kim JY, Park SY, Yoon HS, Cho S, Park HS. Quick and easy correction of a symptomatic pincer nail using a shape memory alloy device. Dermatol Surg. 2013;39(10):1520–6.

18. Nam HM, Kim UK, Park SD, Kim JH, Park K. Correction of pincer nail deformity using dermal grafting. Ann Dermatol. 2011;23 Suppl 3:S299–302.

19. Lin CT, Chen TM. Regarding assisting pincer nail deformity by Haneke's procedure. Dermatol Surg. 2013;39(8):1287–8.

20. Jemec GBE, Kollerup G, Jensen LB, Mogensen S. Nail abnormailities in nondermatologic patients: prevalence and possible role as diagnostic aids. J Am Acad Dermatol. 1995;32(6):977–81.

21. Baran R. The nail in the elderly. Clin Dermatol. 2011;9(1):54–60.

22. Baran R. Nail care in the "golden years" of life. Curr Med Res Opin. 1982;7 Suppl 2:95–7.

23. Lubach D, Cohrs W, Wurzinger R. Incidence of brittle nails. Dermatologica. 1986;172:144–7.

24. Stern DK, Diamantis S, Smith E, Wei H, Gordon M, Muigai W, et al. Water content and other aspects of brittle versus normal fingernails. J Am Acad Dermatol. 2007;57:31–6.

25. Duarte AF, Correia O, Baran R. Nail plate cohesion seems to be water independent. Int J Dermatol. 2009;48:193–5.

26. Forslind B. Biophysical studies on the normal nail. Acta Derm Venereol. 1970;50(3):161–8.

27. Farran L, Ennos AR, Eichhorn SJ. The effect of humidity on fracture properties of human fingernails. J Exp Biol. 2008;211:3677–81.

28. Sasaki M, Kusubata M, Akamatsu H. Biochemical analysis of keratin in the brittle nail. J Invest Dermatol. 2008;128(Suppl 1s):S91.

29. Lubach D, Beckers P. Wet working conditions increase brittleness of nails but do not cause it. Dermatology. 1992;185:120–213.

30. Dimitris R, Daniel CR. Management of simple brittle nails. Dermatol Ther. 2012;25(6):569–73.

31. Shemer A, Daniel CR. Common nail disorders. Clin Dermatol. 2013;31(5):578–86.

32. van de Kerkhof PCM, Pasch MC, Scher RK, Kerscher M, Gieler U, Haneke E, et al. Brittle nail syndrome: a pathogenesis-based approach with a proposed grading system. J Am Acad Dermatol. 2005;53(4):644–51.

33. Zarzour JG, Singh S, Andea A, Cafardi JA. Acrokeratosis paraneoplastica (Bazex syndrome): report of a case associated with small cell lung cancer and a review of the literature. J Radiol Case Rep. 2011;5(7):1–6.

34. Cashman MW, Sloan SB. Nutrition and nail disease. Clin Dermatol. 2010;28(4):420–5.

35. Salem A, Al Mokadem S, Attwa E, Abd El Raoof S, Ebrahim HM, Faheem KT. Nail changes in chronic renal failure patients under haemodialysis. J Eur Acad Dermatol Venereol. 2008;22(11):1326–31.

36. Chao SC, Lee JY. Brittle nails and dyspareunia as first clues to recurrences of malignant glucagonoma. Br J Dermatol. 2002;146(6):1071–4.

37. Geyer A, Scher RK, Uyttendaele H. Brittle nails: pathogenesis and treatment. J Drugs Dermatol. 2003;2(1):48–9.

38. Iorizzo M, Pazzaglia M, Piraccini BM, Tullo S, Tosti A. Brittle nails. J Cosmet Dermatol. 2004;3(3): 138–44.

39. Sparavigna A, Setaro M, Genet M, Frisenda L. *Equisetum arvense* in a new transungual technology improves nail structure and appearance. J Plast Dermatol. 2006;2(1):31–8.

40. Goldstein B, Nasir A, Swick L, van Cleeff M. Clinical evaluation of safety and efficacy of a new topical treatment for onychomycosis. J Drugs Dermatol. 2011;10(10):1186–91.

41. Hochman LG, Scher RK, Meyerson MS. Brittle nails: response to daily biotin supplementation. Cutis. 1993;51(4):303–5.

42. Sherber NS, Hoch AM, Coppola CA, Carter EL, Chang HL, Barsanti FR, et al. Efficacy and safety study of tazarotene cream 0.1 % for the treatment of brittle nail syndrome. Cutis. 2011;87(2): 96–103.

43. Sobera JO, Elewski BE. Onychomycosis. In: Scher RK, Daniel CR, editors. Nails: diagnosis, therapy, surgery. 3rd ed. Philadelphia: Saunders; 2005. p. 123–40.

44. Ghannoum MD, Hajjeh RA, Scher R. A large-scale North American study of fungal isolates from nails: the frequency of onychomycosis, fungal distributions, and antifungal susceptibility patterns. J Am Acad Dermatol. 2000;43:641–8.

45. Elewski B, Charif MA. Prevalence of onychomycosis in patients attending a dermatology clinic in northeastern Ohio for other conditions. Arch Dermatol. 1997;133:1172–3.

46. Thomas J, Jacobson GA, Narkowicz CK, Peterson GM, Burnet H, Sharpe C. Toenail onychomycosis: an important global disease burden. J Clin Pharm Ther. 2010;35(5):497–519.

47. Hay RJ, Baran R. Onychomycosis: a proposed revision of the clinical classification. J Am Acad Dermatol. 2011;65(6):1219–27.

48. Daniel CR, Norton LA, Scher RK. The spectrum of nail disease in patients with human immunodeficiency virus infection. J Am Acad Dermatol. 1992; 27:93–7.

49. Baran R. Proximal subungual Candida onychomycosis: an unusual manifestation of chronic mucocutaneous candidiasis. Br J Dermatol. 1997;137:286–8.

50. Rich P, Elewski B, Scher RK, Pariser D. Diagnosis, clinical implications, complications of onychomycosis. Semin Cutan Med Surg. 2013;32(2 Suppl 1):S5–8.

51. Wilsmann-Theis D, Bieber T, Schmid-Wendtner MH, Wenzel J. New reasons for histopathological nail-clipping examination in the diagnosis of onychomycosis. J Eur Acad Dermatol Venereol. 2011; 25(2):235–7.

52. Gupta AK, Fleckman P, Baran R. Ciclopirox nail lacquer topical solution 8 % in the treatment of toenail onychomycosis. J Am Acad Dermatol. 2000; 43(4 Suppl):S70–80.

53. Baran R, Coquard F. Combination of fluconazole and urea in a nail laquer for treating onychomycosis. J Dermatolog Treat. 2005;16(1):52–5.

54. Elewski BE, Rich P, Pollak R, Pariser DM, Watanabe S, Senda H, et al. Efinaconazole 10 % solution in the treatment of toenail onychomycosis: two phase III multicenter, randomized, double-blind studies. J Am Acad Dermatol. 2013;68(4):600–8.

55. Del Rosso JQ, Reece B, Smith K, Miller T. Efinaconazole 10 % solution: a new topical treatment for onychomycosis: contact sensitization and skin irritation potential. J Clin Aesthet Dermatol. 2013;6(3):20–4.

56. Baker SJ, Zhang YK, Akama T, Lau A, Zhou H, Hernandez V, et al. Discovery of a new boron containing anti-fungal agent, 5-fluoro-1,3-dihydro-1-hydroxy-,1-benzoxaborole (AN2690), for the potential treatment of onychomycosis. J Med Chem. 2006;49(15):4447–50.

57. Elewski BE, Tosti A. Tavaborole for the treatment of onychomycosis. Expert Opin Pharmacother. 2014; 15(10):1439–48.

58. Roberts DR, Taylor WD, Boyle J. Guidelines for treatment of onychomycosis. Br J Dermatol. 2003; 148:402–10.

59. Loo DS. Onychomycosis in the elderly: drug treatment options. Drugs Aging. 2007;24(4):293–302.

60. Lecha M, Effendy I, Feuilhade de Chauvin M, Di Chiacchio N, Baran R. Treatment options—development of consensus guidelines. J Eur Acad Dermatol Venereol. 2005;19 Suppl 1:25–33.

61. Roberts DT, Evans EG. Subungual dermatophytoma complicating dermatophyte onychomycosis. Br J Dermatol. 1998;138(1):189–90.

62. Balfour JA, Faulds D. Terbinafine: a review of its pharmacodynamics and pharmokinetic properties, and therapeutic potential in superficial mycoses. Drugs. 1992;43(2):259–84.

63. Piraccini BM, Sisti A, Tosti A. Long-term followup of toenail onychomycosis caused by dermatophytes after successful treatment with systemic antifungal agents. J Am Acad Dermatol. 2010; 62(3):411–4.

64. Yin Z, Xu J, Luo D. A meta-analysis comparing longterm recurrences of toenail onychomycosis after successful treatment with terbinafine versus itraconazole. J Dermatolog Treat. 2012;23(6):449–52.

65. de Sá DC, Lamas AP, Tosti A. Oral therapy for onychomycosis: an evidence-based review. Am J Clin Dermatol. 2014;15(1):17–36.

66. Gupta AK, Ryder JE, Johnson AM. Cumulative meta-analysis of systemic antifungal agents for the treatment of onychomycosis. Br J Dermatol. 2004; 150:537–44.

67. Gupta AK, Paquet M, Simpson F, Tavakkol A. Terbinafine in the treatment of dermatophyte toenail onychomycosis: a meta-analysis of efficacy for continuous and intermittent regimens. J Eur Acad Dermatol Venereol. 2013;27(3):267–72.

68. Sigurgeirsson B, Billstein S, Rantanen T, Ruzicka T, di Fonzo E, Vermeer BJ, et al. L.I.O.N. Study: efficacy and tolerablility of continuous terbinafine (Lamisil®) compared to intermittent itraconazole in the treatment of toenail onychomycosis. Br J Dermatol. 1999;141 Suppl 56:5–14.

69. Drake LA, Shear NH, Arlette JP, Cloutier R, Danby FW, Elewski BE, et al. Oral terbinafine in the treatment of toenail onychomycosis: North American multicenter trial. J Am Acad Dermatol. 1997; 37(5 Pt 1):740–5.

70. Shapiro LE, Shear NH. Drug interactions: proteins, pumps, and P-450s. J Am Acad Dermatol. 2002; 47(4):467–88.

71. Elewski BE. Mechanism of action of systemic antifungal agents. J Am Acad Dermatol. 1993;28(5 Pt 1): S28–34.

72. Ahmad SR, Singer SJ, Leissa BG. Congestive heart failure associated with itraconazole. Lancet. 2001; 357(9270):1766–7.

73. Onmel (itraconazole) [package insert]. Greensboro, NC: Merz Pharmaceuticals, LLC; 2012.

74. Cathcart S, Cantrell W, Elewski BE. Onychomycosis and diabetes. J Eur Acad Dermatol Venereol. 2009;23(10):1119–22.

75. Gupta AK, Konnikov N, Lynde CW. Single-blind, randomized, prospective study on terbinafine and itraconazole for treatment of dermatophyte toenail onychomycosis in the elderly. J Am Acad Dermatol. 2001;44(3):479–84.

76. Tavakkol A, Fellman S, Kianifard F. Safety and efficacy of oral terbinafine in the treatment of onychomycosis: analysis of the elderly subgroup in Improving Results in ONychomycosis-Concomitant Lamasil and Debridement (IRON-CLAD), an open-label,

randomized trial. Am J Geriatr Pharmacother. 2006; 4(1):1–13.

77. Ortiz AE, Avram MM, Wanner MA. A review of lasers and light for the treatment of onychomycosis. Lasers Surg Med. 2014;46(2):117–24.

78. Hollmig ST, Rahman Z, Henderson MT, Rotatori RM, Gladstone H, Tang JY. Lack of efficacy with 1064-nm neodymium:yttrium-aluminum-garnet laser for the treatment of onychomycosis: a randomized controlled trial. J Am Acad Dermatol. 2014;70(5):911–7.

79. Domínguez-Cherit J, Chanussot-Deprez C, Maria-Sarti H, Fonte-Avalos V, Vega-Memije E, Luis-Montoya P. Nail unit tumors: a study of 234 patients in the dermatology department of the "Dr Manuel Gea González" General Hospital in Mexico City. Dermatol Surg. 2008;34(10):1363–71.

80. Salsache SJ, Orengo IF. Tumors of the nail unit. J Dermatol Surg Oncol. 1992;18(8):691–700.

81. Tosti A, Richert B, Pazzaglia M. Tumors of the nail apparatus. In: Scher RK, Daniel CR, editors. Nails: diagnosis, therapy, surgery. 3rd ed. Philadelphia: Saunders; 2005. p. 195–204.

82. Lin YC, Wu YH, Scher RK. Nail changes and association of osteoarthritis in digital myxoid cyst. Dermatol Surg. 2008;34(3):364–9.

83. Drapé JL, Idy-Peretti I, Goettmann S, Salon A, Abimelec P, Guérin-Surville H, et al. MR imaging of digital mucoid cysts. Radiology. 1996;200(2): 531–6.

84. De Berker DA, Lawrence CM. Treatment of myxoid cysts. Dermatol Surg. 2001;27(3):296–9.

85. Epstein E. A simple technique for managing digital mucous cysts. Arch Dermatol. 1979;115(11): 1315–6.

86. Van Geertruyden J, Lorea P, Goldschmidt D, de Fontaine S, Schuind F, Kinnen L, et al. Glomus tumors of the hand: a retrospective study of 51 cases. J Hand Surg Br. 1996;21(2):257–60.

87. Richert B, Lecerf P, Caucanas M, André J. Nail tumors. Clin Dermatol. 2013;31(5):602–17.

88. Jablon M, Horowitz A, Bernstein DA. Magnetic resonance imaging of a glomus tumor of the fingertip. J Hand Surg Am. 1990;15(3):507–9.

89. Drapé JL, Idy-Peretti I, Goettmann S, Guérin-Surville H, Bittoun J. Standard and high resolution magnetic resonance imaging of glomus tumors of toes and fingertips. J Am Acad Dermatol. 1996;35(4): 550–5.

90. Richert B, Baghaie M. Medical imaging and MRI in nail disorders: report of 119 cases and review. Dermatol Ther. 2002;15(2):159–64.

91. Lin YC, Hsiao PF, Wu YH, Sun FJ, Scher RK. Recurrent digital glomus tumor: analysis of 75 cases. Dermatol Surg. 2010;36(9):1396–400.

92. Lecerf P, Richert B, Theunis A, André J. A retrospective study of squamous cell carcinoma of the nail unit diagnosed in a Belgian general hospital over a 15-year period. J Am Acad Dermatol. 2013;69(2):253–61.

93. Riddel C, Rashid R, Thomas V. Ungual and periungual human papillomavirus-associated squamous cell carcinoma: a review. J Am Acad Dermatol. 2011;64(6):1147–53.

94. Attiyeh FF, Shah J, Booher RJ, Knapper WH. Subungual squamous cell carcinoma. JAMA. 1979;241(3):262–3.

95. Hale LR, Dawber RP. Subungual squamous cell carcinoma presenting with minimal nail changes: a factor in delayed diagnosis? Australas J Dermatol. 1998;39(2):86–8.

96. Zaiac MN, Weiss E. Mohs micrographic surgery of the nail unit and squamous cell carcinoma. Dermatol Surg. 2001;27(3):246–51.

97. Lumpkin LR, Rosen T, Tschen JA. Subungual squamous cell carcinoma. J Am Acad Dermatol. 1984;11(4 Pt 2):734–8.

98. Dika E, Piraccini BM, Balestri R, Vaccari S, Misciali C, Patrizi A, et al. Mohs surgery for squamous cell carcinoma of the nail: report of 15 cases. Our experience and a long-term follow-up. Br J Dermatol. 2012;167(6):1310–4.

99. Banfield CC, Redburn JC, Dawber RPR. The incidence and prognosis of nail apparatus melanoma: a retrospective study of 105 patients in four English regions. Br J Dermatol. 1998;139(2):276–9.

100. Blessing K, Kernohan NM, Park KGM. Subungual malignant melanoma: clinicopathologic features of 100 cases. Histopathology. 1991;19(5):425–9.

101. Finley RK, Driscoll DL, Blumenson LE, Karakousis CP. Subungual melanoma: an eighteen-year review. Surgery. 1994;116(1):96–100.

102. Kato T, Suetake T, Sugiyama Y, Tabata N, Tagami H. Epidemiology and prognosis of subungual melanoma in 34 Japanese patients. Br J Dermatol. 1996;134(3):383–7.

103. Thai KE, Young R, Sinclair RD. Nail apparatus melanoma. Australas J Dermatol. 2001;42(2):71–81.

104. Thomas L, Zook EG, Haneke E, Drapé JL, Baran R, Kreusch JF. Tumors of the nail apparatus and adjacent tissues. In: Baran R, de Berker DAR, Holzbert M, Thomas L, editors. Baran & Dawber's diseases of the nails and their management. 4th ed. Oxford: Blackwell; 2012. p. 637–743.

105. Cohen T, Busam KJ, Patel A, Brady MS. Subungal melanoma: management considerations. Am J Surg. 2008;195(2):244–8.

106. Quinn MJ, Thompson JE, Crotty K, McCarthy WH, Coates AS. Subungual melanoma of the hand. J Hand Surg Am. 1996;21(3):506–11.

107. Tan KB, Moncrieff M, Thompson JF, McCarthy SW, Shaw HM, Quinn MJ, et al. Subungual melanoma: a study of 124 cases highlighting features of early lesions, potential pitfalls in diagnosis, and guidelines for histologic reporting. Am J Surg Pathol. 2007; 31(12):1902–12.

108. Nguyen JT, Bakri K, Nguyen EC, Johnson CH, Moran SL. Surgical management of subungual melanoma: Mayo Clinic experience of 124 cases. Ann Plast Surg. 2013;71(4):346–54.
109. Saida T. Heterogeneity of the site of origin of malignant melanoma in ungual areas: "Subungual" malignant melanoma may be a misnomer. Br J Dermatol. 1992;126(5):529.
110. Banfield CC, Dawber RPR. Nail melanoma: a review of the literature with recommendations to improve patient management. Br J Dermatol. 1999;141(4): 628–32.
111. Saida T, Ohshima Y. Clinical and histopathologic characteristics of early lesions of subungual malignant melanoma. Cancer. 1989;63(3):556–60.
112. Levit EK, Kagen MH, Scher RK, Grossman M, Altman E. The ABC rule for clinical detection of subungal melanoma. J Am Acad Dermatol. 2000; 42(2 Pt 1):269–74.
113. Baran R, Kechijian P. Hutchinson's sign: a reappraisal. J Am Acad Dermatol. 1996;34(1):87–90.
114. Shulka VK, Hughes LE. Differential diagnosis of subungual melanoma from a surgical point of view. Br J Surg. 1989;76(11):1156–60.
115. André J, Moulonguet I, Goettmann-Bonvallot S. In situ amelanotic melanomia of the nail unit mimicking lichen planus: report of 3 cases. Arch Dermatol. 2010;146(4):418–21.
116. Martin DE, English JC, Goitz RJ. Subungual malignant melanoma. J Hand Surg Am. 2011;36(4):704–7.

Hormonal Regulation and Systemic Signals of Skin Aging

Gregory W. Charville and Anne Lynn S. Chang

Significance of Systemic Signals in Skin Aging

Physicians have long appreciated that skin can manifest signs of systemic illness [1]. In the fourth century B.C., Hippocrates classified skin diseases as "local" or "constitutional" [2]. Those in the latter class were attributed to bodily humors making an outward display of their "distemper" [3]. Although we no longer think of skin disease in terms of imbalances of humors, Hippocrates' thinking in many ways foreshadowed our current understanding of the contribution of systemic signals to skin pathology. Indeed, we now appreciate that skin lesions commonly reflect abnormalities in circulating factors in the setting of oncologic, autoimmune, endocrine, and nutritional disorders.

Among these circulating factors, hormones represent a broad class of regulatory chemicals conveyed by tissue fluids to stimulate signaling responses at distant targets. Because of their capacity for action at a distance, hormones are linked to skin pathology that is diffuse or poorly localized, as in the case of xeroderma due to hypothyroidism or hyperpigmentation due to adrenal insufficiency [1]. Aging leads to a number of changes to skin throughout the body, including diminished dermal and epidermal thickness [4], altered collagen and elastic fiber organization [5], poor wound-healing [6], and a decline in apocrine and eccrine gland frequency and function [7]. The question therefore arises as to whether the generalized pathology associated with skin aging is due to changes in systemic hormone signals. In this chapter, we discuss the evidence for hormonal regulation of phenomena linked to aging in skin (summarized in Table 1), and consider the opportunities for clinical application of hormonal modification to promote skin health during aging.

Basic Studies of Hormones in Skin Aging

Given the potential for manipulation of the course of skin aging by systemic signals, there has been an effort to study these signals in a controlled context, allowing for thorough analyses of hormone levels and preliminary tests of pharmaceutical interventions to reverse aging phenotypes. One method to test the role of the systemic milieu on skin aging involves experiments in which the circulation of old and young animals are

G.W. Charville (✉)
Departments of Dermatology and Pathology,
Stanford University School of Medicine,
450 Broadway St., Redwood City, CA 94063, USA
e-mail: gwc@stanford.edu

A.L.S. Chang, M.D.
Assistant Professor, Department of Dermatology,
Stanford University School of Medicine,
450 Broadway Street, MC5334,
Redwood City, CA 94063, USA

© Springer International Publishing Switzerland 2015
A.L.S. Chang (ed.), *Advances in Geriatric Dermatology*, DOI 10.1007/978-3-319-18380-0_4

Table 1 Summary of hormonal changes involved in skin aging

Hormone pathway	Direction of change with age	Associated phenotypes
IGF	↓	Sebum production, increased pore size, epithelial disorganization
NF-κB	↑	Atrophy, epidermal senescence, reduced cell proliferation
Estrogen	↓	Atrophy, impaired wound-healing, xerosis, wrinkling, abnormal pigmentation
Wnt	↑	HFSC senescence, decline in HFSC number, atrophy, impaired wound healing
Testosterone	↓	Decreased elasticity, atrophy, low epidermal water content, hair loss
BMP/NFATc1	↑	Impaired HFSC activation, poor hair regrowth
TGF-β	↓	Reduced collagen content, impaired wound healing
Glucocorticoids	↑	Decreased dermal cellularity, atrophy, poor wound healing, reduced collagen content, flattened rete ridges, decreased dermal fibroblast proliferation

surgically linked [8]. In these so-called parabiosis experiments, tissues from a linked heterochronic pair consisting of one old and one young mouse are compared to tissues of control isochronic pairs consisting of two young mice or two old mice. Thus, the effect of a young systemic milieu on the aged tissue phenotype and the effect of an aged systemic milieu on the young tissue phenotype can be evaluated.

In early experiments employing this technique, the regeneration of aged skeletal muscle and hepatic tissue in response to acute injury were enhanced by exposure to a young systemic environment [9]. In the brain, parabiosis studies demonstrated that neurogenesis in young mice is impaired by hormones present in the circulation of old mice [10]. Although the effects of parabiosis on skin aging have not been extensively explored, recent investigation of the impact of age on mouse hair follicle regeneration revealed enhancement of the in vitro colony-forming potential of hair follicle stem cells (HFSCs) from aged mice following heterochronic parabiosis [11].

In exploring the mechanisms by which an aging systemic milieu can suppress the regenerative potential of young tissue, an excess of Wnt signaling activity has been identified in aged serum [8]. That pathologic Wnt signaling plays a role in mammalian aging was supported by the observation that mutant *klotho* mice, which display phenotypes of precocious aging, also have abnormally high levels of circulating Wnt [12]. This exaggerated Wnt signaling can be attributed to the loss of a Wnt inhibitory factor encoded by the *klotho* allele. Skin atrophy and impaired wound-healing are among the aging phenotypes of *klotho* mutants [13], suggesting that Wnt is a circulating factor that can dictate the functional phenotypes of aging skin. Indeed, mice engineered to express Wnt at supraphysiologic levels display markers of senescence in skin cells akin to what is observed in *klotho* mutants [12]. Excess Wnt seemed to be particularly harmful to HFSCs, which were depleted from the follicle in mice lacking *klotho*. Human klotho exhibits 86 % amino-acid sequence similarity with the mouse protein. Although there are no studies examining the specific role of klotho in human skin aging, a recent population-based association study has suggested a correlation between functionally distinct *KLOTHO* alleles and both life expectancy and longevity [14]. Understanding whether these *KLOTHO* variants predict, or even determine, characteristics of human skin aging will be an important area for future investigation.

Tissue-specific stem cells may play an especially important role in the manifestation of skin aging phenotypes. This association arises from the observation that aging often reflects impairment of homeostatic tissue repair, which is generally the job of resident adult stem cells [15]. Furthermore, stem cells are uniquely sensitive to hormonal growth factors that are commonly dysregulated in aged animals [16]. In addition to their sensitivity to increased Wnt signaling, HFSCs show an age-dependent decline in hair follicle regeneration that is linked to their overstimulation by bone morphogenetic proteins (BMPs) [11]. In studies by Fuchs and colleagues, increases in the expression of *Bmp2*, *Bmp4*, and *Bmp6* in the skin of aged mice were found to cause abnormal activation of the transcription factor NFATc1. The dysregulated BMP-NFATc1 axis impairs the activation of aged HFSCs in response to follicle depilation. Treatment of old mice with systemic inhibitors of BMP or NFATc1 returned HFSCs' youthful capacity for hair regrowth, indicating that alterations in BMP-NFATc1 signaling caused reversible impairment of aged HFSCs.

The influence of BMP signaling on the function of skin stem cells during aging may relate in part to its regulation by hormonal TGF-β signaling. In healthy, young skin, TGF-β normally inhibits the repressive effects of BMP signaling through the activation of *Tmeff1* [17]. In aged skin, however, TGF-β levels are markedly reduced, and this reduction is associated with a decrease in the level of type I collagen production [18]. Reducing the level of TGF-β in young skin is also sufficient to reduce local collagen content. This effect of TGF-β may be driven by a synergistic interaction with connective tissue growth factor (CTGF), which augments the increased expression of collagen induced by TGF-β and also decreases during aging [19]. Although TGF-β levels have not been linked directly to the decline in skin stem cell function during aging, changes in the efficiency of skin wound healing seen in aged mammals have been attributed to low TGF-β. These studies revealed a decline in expression of all three TGF-β isoforms within regenerating wounds of aged mice [20]. In agreement with these findings, analyses of mutants lacking functional TGF-β1 [21], TGF-β3 [22], or TGF-β receptor type II [23], revealed impaired wound healing, including reduced collagen deposition and poor wound contraction. Whether pharmacologic stimulation of TGF-β signaling is sufficient to improve wound healing in the context of aging is yet to be studied. Nonetheless, the addition of

TGF-β3 to wounds increases the rate of healing even in young animals [24]. Also of note, exogenous erythropoietin accelerates wound healing by inducing expression of TGF-β1 [25]. In humans, exposure to ultraviolet radiation, known for inducing aging-associated skin damage, impairs TGF-β signaling and thus causes a reduction in collagen expression [26, 27]. Decreased epidermal TGF-β signaling may also have a role independent of ultraviolet radiation in intrinsic skin aging [28]. Although stimulation of TGF-β signaling in human skin fibroblasts in vitro is sufficient to induce collagen expression [29], future clinical trials are required to evaluate the effects of exogenous TGF-β on human skin. An important consideration in the therapeutic modulation of TGF-β signaling for enhanced wound healing or the prevention of skin aging, however, is the concern that excess activation of this pathway may contribute to the formation of hypertrophic scarring or fibrosis [30–32].

Changes in the systemic milieu during aging will by definition have the potential to impact tissues throughout the body. Therefore, it stands to reason that a broader survey of age-dependent pathology will identify shared mechanisms that point to hormonal dysregulation. Employing this logic, Chang and colleagues performed an elegant analysis of genome-wide mRNA expression data from 365 microarrays encompassing nine different human and mouse tissues, including skin, to determine which *cis*-regulatory motifs were over-represented among those genes for which expression changes significantly with age [33]. Remarkably, the motif most strongly associated with age-dependent gene expression changes was that of NF-κB, a transcription factor responsible for conveying the message of numerous hormonal signals. Among the known regulators of NF-κB activity are tumor necrosis factor alpha (TNF-α), interleukin 1 beta (IL-1β), epidermal growth factor (EGF), fibroblast growth factor (FGF), platelet-derived growth factor (PDGF), progesterone, and glucocorticoids [34]. The implication of this finding is that increased NF-κB-dependent transcription is responsible, at least in part, for the aging phenotype of skin, among other tissues. To test this model, NF-κB was inhibited in aged skin by expressing a dominant-negative NF-κB allele [33, 35]. Of the 414 genes that showed age-dependent changes in expression in mouse skin, 225 returned to the level observed in young mice upon inhibition of NF-κB. Abrogating NF-κB in aged skin also increased skin thickness and epidermal cell proliferation, while decreasing the amount of cell senescence normally observed during aging. Although elevated NF-κB signaling in aged skin has yet to be linked to signaling by a particular hormone, previous studies have shown dysregulation of TNF-α [36, 37], PDGF [20], FGF [38, 39], and cortisol [40] levels during aging.

Clinical Studies of Hormonal Regulation of Aging in Skin

Among human hormones thought to be involved in skin aging, the sex hormones have received the bulk of attention in clinical studies. The prevalence of studies examining the effects of estrogens and androgens may be attributed to a well-understood phenomenon of sex hormone reduction in both genders with age, and to the popularity of sex hormone replacement therapy. In women, menopause marks the cessation of estrogen production by the ovaries, and a consequent drop in circulating hormone levels. Estradiol, the predominant estrogen during reproductive years in terms of both estrogenic activity and absolute serum levels, decreases by 80 % during menopause [41]. Menopause thus mimics a natural loss-of-function experiment for studying the role of estrogens in skin biology. Phenotypes of aging skin linked to declining estrogen levels during menopause include atrophy, xeroderma, wrinkling, fragility, and poor wound-healing [42].

Clinically, many of these phenotypes are abrogated with estrogen replacement. Following menopause, the dermal collagen content declines by 1–2 % per year [43], and this decline correlates better with age relative to menopause than with absolute age [44]. In two randomized, placebo-controlled studies, estrogen replacement for 6–12 months increased the skin collagen content of postmenopausal women [45, 46].

Estrogen replacement also led to a 33 % increase in skin thickness over a period of 12 months of therapy [47]. Skin wrinkling and laxity are two phenomena of aging thought to reflect a loss of tissue elasticity. Bolognia et al. identified degenerative changes in the elastic fibers of menopausal women [48], and subsequent studies revealed enhanced size and concentration of elastic fibers with estrogen replacement [49, 50]. Others have used computerized suction devices to measure the extensibility of skin in postmenopausal women receiving estrogen therapy or placebo, and have shown consistently that estrogens prevent the increase in skin extensibility, and decrease in elasticity, normally seen during menopause [51, 52]. Unfortunately, in vitro studies have not easily translated into clearly effective treatments for aging-related skin pathologies. To date, small clinical trials of topical estrogen cream on skin aging parameters such as rhytides have not consistently demonstrated significant effects, and hence this treatment modality is not the standard of care in general dermatologic practice [53, 54].

Estrogen also seems to have beneficial effects on skin wound healing. In one study, men and women treated with transdermal estrogen at the site of a punch biopsy had faster wound repair and increased wound collagen levels [55]. Estrogen replacement also prevented the onset of chronic venous stasis or pressure ulcers [56]. The beneficial effects of estrogen on wound healing may relate to stimulation of TGF-β secretion at the site of the wound [57], and to the suppression of pro-inflammatory macrophage migration inhibitory factor [58]. Despite its overall favorable impact on aging phenotypes in skin, the regular use of oral estrogen replacement therapy remains limited by its association with increased risk of venous thromboembolism, stroke, heart disease, and breast cancer [59, 60].

Selective estrogen receptor modulators (SERMs), which both activate and block estrogen receptors, have also been studied for their effects on human skin. In human skin fibroblasts, collagen biosynthesis has been observed to increase in response to oral raloxifene, a SERM [61]. In a small study in postmenopausal women, raloxifene has also been reported to improve skin elasticity [62]. Whether these improvements are clinically significant and whether the risk–benefit ratio of SERMs is favorable for antiaging indications remains to be determined.

Estrogen depletion at menopause is thought to explain the accelerated rate of skin aging, especially in terms of skin atrophy, observed in females as compared to males [63]. However, men too undergo a so-called "andropause" associated with a decline in testosterone levels with age [64]. Many of the age-related changes associated with postmenopausal estrogen reduction, such as decreases in skin thickness and elasticity, have also been linked to low testosterone [65]. Likewise, testosterone replacement can lead to rejuvenation of the skin of aged men, inducing increased epidermal thickness and dermal mucopolysaccharide content [66]. Perhaps the most recognizable effect of androgens is their regulation of hair growth. In contrast to the involvement of increased androgen signaling in the androgenic alopecia seen in younger men, aged men undergo a separate process of hair loss associated with dwindling testosterone levels [67]. Women also exhibit beneficial hair regrowth in response to androgen replacement therapies [68]. Interestingly, the diverse effect of androgens on hair follicle function may reflect anatomical heterogeneity in follicle hormone receptor expression [69, 70]. Thus, the age-dependent decline in androgen levels is predicted to manifest as a variable hair loss dictated in part by positional differences in androgen sensitivity.

Glucocorticoids represent another class of steroid hormone for which there have been ample clinical studies owing to the prevalence of glucocorticoid-based treatments of dermatologic and non-dermatologic conditions. The association of glucocorticoid signaling with aging stems from the striking similarity between the phenotypes observed in aged individuals and in individuals with glucocorticoid excess. It is now known that both aging and glucocorticoid excess cause dermal and epidermal thinning [71, 72], flattening of the rete ridges at the dermal–epidermal junction [73, 74], poor wound healing [75, 76], and reduced collagen content [77–80]. These observations have led to the hypothesis that age-related skin pathology can be attributed to an increase in glucocorticoid signaling.

As mentioned, some have attributed an excess of glucocorticoid signaling in adults to elevated circulating cortisol [40]. However, in these studies of healthy human volunteers, significant variation in cortisol levels were noted, and a subset of individuals had a decrease in cortisol levels with age. Given this discrepancy, some have argued that excess glucocorticoid signaling is instead related to local enzymatic regulation of cortisol availability [81]. In support of this model, investigators found that the expression of 11-β-hydroxysteroid dehydrogenase type 1 (11β-HSD1) in the skin of aged humans and mice is higher than that observed in young subjects. 11β-HSD1 is a cellular oxoreductase that converts cortisone to cortisol. Additional studies have shown that 11β-HSD1 expression is also increased in photo-exposed relative to photo-protected skin, implying that this mechanism may account also for skin photoaging [82]. Remarkably, genetic loss of 11β-HSD1 leads to reduced skin atrophy and increased skin collagen content in aged mice [81]. Likewise, application of a small-molecule inhibitor of 11β-HSD1 to the skin of aged mice enhances the rate of wound healing. Thus, excess glucocorticoid signaling appears to be a clinically tractable feature of skin aging.

Recently, techniques for global gene expression analysis have been used to study the molecular changes undergone by skin during aging that are likely to underlie the phenotypes we associate with aged skin. Although these studies fundamentally reflect changes within the skin cells themselves, it follows that these intrinsic characteristics reflect alterations in the systemic environment, and therefore may be used to shed light on the mechanisms by which systemic signals affect skin physiology during aging. One such study examined global gene expression using RNA sequencing in five young (age <30 years) and five old (age >50 years) subjects before and after treatment of skin with broadband light [83]. With this study design, investigators were able to identify changes in gene expression patterns associated with aging and those associated with rejuvenation, or a return to youthful levels, induced by treatment with broadband light. Among the genes for which expression was rejuvenated by broadband light, there were a number associated with the intracellular transduction of hormonal signaling.

One of these genes, *IGF1R*, is the tyrosine kinase receptor for insulin-like growth factor 1 and 2. IGF1/2 signaling is known to be a critical regulator of aging that is conserved among humans and model organisms. Notably, disabling mutations in the *C. elegans* homolog of *IGF1R*, *daf-2*, were the first to be associated with lifespan extension [84]. Regulation of IGF signaling has since been shown to influence lifespan in yeast, flies, and mice [85]. Though controlled manipulations of IGF signaling have not yet been studied in humans, functional mutations of *IGF1R* that generate decreased IGF signaling have been identified in exceptionally long-lived individuals [86]. Furthermore, circulating levels of IGF-1 are lower in the offspring of human centenarians compared to age-matched offspring controls [87]. The correlation with decreased IGF signaling and tissue youthfulness is similar in human skin, where broadband light reverses the elevated expression of *IGFR1* seen in aged subjects [83]. Interestingly, in one study of otherwise healthy young women (aged 22–41), increased IGF-1 levels in the skin were correlated with poor cosmetic characteristics such as increased facial pore area, sebum production, and epithelial disorganization [88]. The connection between IGF signaling and skin aging has been reinforced in multiple subsequent genome-wide association studies. In a case-control genome-wide association study of aged individuals who lack global features of skin aging, skin youthfulness was associated with a single-nucleotide polymorphism near *EDEM1* [89], the expression of which correlates with expression of *IGF1* in a mouse model of longevity [90]. In a similar genome-wide association study of skin aging in middle-aged women, a polymorphism that influences expression of *FBXO40*, a regulator of IGF signaling, was noted [91]. Taken together, these studies hint strongly at a role for IGF signaling in the progression of human skin aging, although the precise mechanisms by which alterations in IGF signaling lead to aging phenotypes remain to be elucidated.

Studies of gene expression in human skin have also added support for the aforementioned role of NF-κB in the aging process. In the group of genes exhibiting photo-reversible changes in expression with age, targets of NF-κB are significantly overrepresented [83]. It should be noted, however, that interactions between NF-κB and IGF signaling have been identified, and that the observation of age-related alterations in these pathways may therefore reflect their interdependence.

Future Directions

Advances in the study and clinical application of hormones and signaling pathways in skin aging will be dictated in large part by the development of new technologies. Among these technologies, improvements in the speed and accuracy of nucleic acid sequencing, and the related reduction in sequencing costs, will enable a broadening of sequencing studies. Although initial studies involving relatively small numbers of sequenced subjects have shed much light on the role of specific signaling pathways in skin aging, expansion of these data sets will allow us to determine how variation in hormonal signals influence aging at the level of individuals. Such studies would contribute to our currently limited understanding of aging heterogeneity—how the process of aging manifests uniquely in each subject. Clinically, more individualized data would allow intervention to be tailored to the needs of a specific patient. For instance, one patient may benefit more from estrogen replacement, another from BMP-NFAT suppression. Eventually, routine testing of patients may involve genome and RNA sequencing from a small skin biopsy.

Initial efforts to sequence the human genome identified numerous so-called "orphan" receptors, which were predicted on the basis of sequence to function as receptors, but which did not have a known ligand. Though the intervening years have seen the "adoption" of hundreds of such receptors, many orphans remain. Recent advances in techniques for determination of receptor structure, particularly in the case of transmembrane receptors, offer a new avenue for the prospective identification of ligands. Because previous screening approaches lacked the sensitivity to detect subtle or unexpected downstream responses [92], new analytical technologies including low-input RNA sequencing or mass spectrometry offer new opportunities for ligand screening. The likelihood that select orphan receptors have roles in skin biology that are relevant to age-related pathology makes this an interesting direction for future study.

Given that stem cell populations mediate many of the effects of age-associated hormonal changes in skin, future advances will benefit from a recent exponential increase in our understanding of skin stem cell biology. New insight into the identity of stem cells in the epidermis and hair follicle have allowed for novel methods to prospectively purify stem cell populations from mouse and human tissue. These isolation techniques enable unprecedented studies of the molecular mechanisms of stem cell-mediated maintenance of skin homeostasis. Future application of these techniques for comparison of stem cell characteristics in young and aged subjects will indicate specifically how skin stem cells are affected by systemic signals in aged individuals. As our knowledge of skin stem cells has grown, so has our ability to manipulate these cells ex vivo for clinical applications. If these cells can be grown in the laboratory, studies involving manipulation of hormonal signaling can be achieved much more efficiently and in a controlled setting. These studies could also be done in a patient-specific manner. Importantly, the successful ex vivo growth of skin stem cells will likely rely on a reconstitution of the hormonal milieu that these cells encounter in vivo. Techniques for efficient growth of stem cells will enable high-throughput screens of functional readouts of hormone signals, including combinatorial screens that look for interactions between hormonal signaling pathways. The most exciting promise of our expanding toolbox for manipulation of skin stem cells is of course the use of these cells for clinical repair of damaged or degenerated tissue. Insight into hormonal regulation of skin stem cell behavior may advance techniques for promoting stem cell engraftment, survival, and self-renewal during transplantation.

References

1. Rigopoulos D, Larios G, Katsambas A. Skin signs of systemic diseases. Clin Dermatol. 2011;29:531–40.
2. Jackson R. Historical outline of attempts to classify skin diseases. Can Med Assoc J. 1977;116:1165–8.
3. Liddell K. Hippocrates of Cos (460–377 bc). Clin Exp Dermatol. 2000;25:86–8.
4. Branchet MC, Boisnic S, Frances C, Robert AM. Skin thickness changes in normal aging skin. Gerontology. 1990;36:28–35.
5. Fenske NA, Lober CW. Structural and functional changes of normal aging skin. J Am Acad Dermatol. 1986;15:571–85.
6. Fenske NA, Conard CB. Aging skin. Am Fam Physician. 1988;37:219–30.
7. Kurban RS, Bhawan J. Histologic changes in skin associated with aging. J Dermatol Surg Oncol. 1990;16:908–14.
8. Brack AS, Conboy MJ, Roy S, Lee M, Kuo CJ, Keller C, et al. Increased Wnt signaling during aging alters muscle stem cell fate and increases fibrosis. Science. 2007;317:807–10.
9. Conboy IM, Conboy MJ, Wagers AJ, Girma ER, Weissman IL, Rando TA. Rejuvenation of aged progenitor cells by exposure to a young systemic environment. Nature. 2005;433:760–4.
10. Villeda SA, Luo J, Mosher KI, Zou B, Britschgi M, Bieri G, et al. The ageing systemic milieu negatively regulates neurogenesis and cognitive function. Nature. 2011;477:90–4.
11. Keyes BE, Segal JP, Heller E, Lien WH, Chang CY, Guo X, et al. Nfatc1 orchestrates aging in hair follicle stem cells. Proc Natl Acad Sci U S A. 2013;110: E4950–9.
12. Liu H, Fergusson MM, Castilho RM, Liu J, Cao L, Chen J, et al. Augmented Wnt signaling in a mammalian model of accelerated aging. Science. 2007;317:803–6.
13. Kuro-o M, Matsumura Y, Aizawa H, Kawaguchi H, Suga T, Utsugi T, et al. Mutation of the mouse klotho gene leads to a syndrome resembling ageing. Nature. 1997;390:45–51.
14. Arking DE, Krebsova A, Macek Sr M, Macek Jr M, Arking A, Mian IS, et al. Association of human aging with a functional variant of klotho. Proc Natl Acad Sci U S A. 2002;99:856–61.
15. Rando TA. Stem cells, ageing and the quest for immortality. Nature. 2006;441:1080–6.
16. Liu L, Rando TA. Manifestations and mechanisms of stem cell aging. J Cell Biol. 2011;193:257–66.

17. Oshimori N, Fuchs E. Paracrine TGF-β signaling counterbalances BMP-mediated repression in hair follicle stem cell activation. Cell Stem Cell. 2012; 10:63–75.

18. Quan T, Shao Y, He T, Voorhees JJ, Fisher GJ. Reduced expression of connective tissue growth factor (CTGF/CCN2) mediates collagen loss in chronologically aged human skin. J Invest Dermatol. 2010;130: 415–24.

19. Chujo S, Shirasaki F, Kawara S, Inagaki Y, Kinbara T, Inaoki M, et al. Connective tissue growth factor causes persistent proalpha2(I) collagen gene expression induced by transforming growth factor-beta in a mouse fibrosis model. J Cell Physiol. 2005;203: 447–56.

20. Ashcroft GS, Horan MA, Ferguson MWJ. The effects of ageing on wound healing: immunolocalisation of growth factors and their receptors in a murine incisional model. J Anat. 1997;190:351–65.

21. Brown RL, Ormsby I, Doetschman TC, Greenhalgh DG. Wound healing in the transforming growth factor-beta-deficient mouse. Wound Repair Regen. 1995;3:25–36.

22. Le M, Naridze R, Morrison J, Biggs LC, Rhea L, Schutte BC, et al. Transforming growth factor beta 3 is required for excisional wound repair in vivo. PLoS One. 2012;7:e48040.

23. Martinez-Ferrer M, Afshar-Sherif AR, Uwamariya C, de Crombrugghe B, Davidson JM, Bhowmick NA. Dermal transforming growth factor-? Responsiveness mediates wound contraction and epithelial closure. Am J Pathol. 2010;176:98–107.

24. Wu L, Siddiqui A, Morris DE, Cox DA, Roth SI, Mustoe TA. Transforming growth factor beta 3 (TGF beta 3) accelerates wound healing without alteration of scar prominence. Histologic and competitive reverse-transcription-polymerase chain reaction studies. Arch Surg. 1997;1960(132):753–60.

25. Siebert N, Xu W, Grambow E, Zechner D, Vollmar B. Erythropoietin improves skin wound healing and activates the TGF-β signaling pathway. Lab Invest. 2011; 91:1753–65.

26. Quan T, He T, Kang S, Voorhees JJ, Fisher GJ. Ultraviolet irradiation alters transforming growth factor beta/smad pathway in human skin in vivo. J Invest Dermatol. 2002;119:499–506.

27. Quan T, He T, Kang S, Voorhees JJ, Fisher GJ. Solar ultraviolet irradiation reduces collagen in photoaged human skin by blocking transforming growth factor-beta type II receptor/Smad signaling. Am J Pathol. 2004;165:741–51.

28. Han K-H, Choi HR, Won CH, Chung JH, Cho KH, Eun HC, et al. Alteration of the TGF-beta/SMAD pathway in intrinsically and UV-induced skin aging. Mech Ageing Dev. 2005;126:560–7.

29. Chen SJ, Yuan W, Mori Y, Levenson A, Trojanowska M, Varga J. Stimulation of type I collagen transcription in human skin fibroblasts by TGF-beta: involvement of Smad 3. J Invest Dermatol. 1999;112:49–57.

30. Schmid P, Itin P, Cherry G, Bi C, Cox DA. Enhanced expression of transforming growth factor-beta type I and type II receptors in wound granulation tissue and hypertrophic scar. Am J Pathol. 1998;152:485–93.

31. Ghahary A, Shen YJ, Scott PG, Gong Y, Tredget EE. Enhanced expression of mRNA for transforming growth factor-beta, type I and type III procollagen in human post-burn hypertrophic scar tissues. J Lab Clin Med. 1993;122:465–73.

32. Zhang K, Garner W, Cohen L, Rodriguez J, Phan S. Increased types I and III collagen and transforming growth factor-beta 1 mRNA and protein in hypertrophic burn scar. J Invest Dermatol. 1995;104:750–4.

33. Adler AS, Sinha S, Kawahara TL, Zhang JY, Segal E, Chang HY. Motif module map reveals enforcement of aging by continual NF-kappaB activity. Genes Dev. 2007;21:3244–57.

34. Delfino F, Walker WH. Hormonal regulation of the NF-κB signaling pathway. Mol Cell Endocrinol. 1999;157:1–9.

35. Adler AS, Kawahara TLA, Segal E, Chang HY. Reversal of aging by NFkappaB blockade. Cell Cycle. 2008;7:556–9.

36. Kirwan JP, Krishnan RK, Weaver JA, Del Aguila LF, Evans WJ. Human aging is associated with altered TNF-alpha production during hyperglycemia and hyperinsulinemia. Am J Physiol Endocrinol Metab. 2001;281:E1137–43.

37. Gupta S, Chiplunkar S, Kim C, Yel L, Gollapudi S. Effect of age on molecular signaling of TNF-alpha-induced apoptosis in human lymphocytes. Mech Ageing Dev. 2003;124:503–9.

38. Chakkalakal JV, Jones KM, Basson MA, Brack AS. The aged niche disrupts muscle stem cell quiescence. Nature. 2012;490:355–60.

39. Komi-Kuramochi A, Kawano M, Oda Y, Asada M, Suzuki M, Oki J, et al. Expression of fibroblast growth factors and their receptors during full-thickness skin wound healing in young and aged mice. J Endocrinol. 2005;186:273–89.

40. Lupien SJ, de Leon M, de Santi S, Convit A, Tarshish C, Nair NP, et al. Cortisol levels during human aging predict hippocampal atrophy and memory deficits. Nat Neurosci. 1998;1:69–73.

41. Yen SSC. The biology of menopause. J Reprodin Med Obstet Gynecol. 1977;18:287–96.

42. Hall G, Phillips TJ. Estrogen and skin: the effects of estrogen, menopause, and hormone replacement therapy on the skin. J Am Acad Dermatol. 2005;53: 555–68.

43. Brincat M, Kabalan S, Studd JW, Moniz CF, de Trafford J, Montgomery J. A study of the decrease of skin collagen content, skin thickness, and bone mass in the postmenopausal woman. Obstet Gynecol. 1987;70:840–5.

44. Brincat M, Moniz CJ, Studd JW, Darby A, Magos A, Emburey G, et al. Long-term effects of the menopause and sex hormones on skin thickness. Br J Obstet Gynaecol. 1985;92:256–9.

45. Sauerbronn AV, Fonseca AM, Bagnoli VR, Saldiva PH, Pinotti JA. The effects of systemic hormonal replacement therapy on the skin of postmenopausal women. Int J Gynaecol Obstet. 2000;68:35–41.

46. Castelo-Branco C, Duran M, González-Merlo J. Skin collagen changes related to age and hormone replacement therapy. Maturitas. 1992;15:113–9.

47. Maheux R, Naud F, Rioux M, Grenier R, Lemay A, Guy J, et al. A randomized, double-blind, placebo-controlled study on the effect of conjugated estrogens on skin thickness. Am J Obstet Gynecol. 1994;170: 642–9.

48. Bolognia JL, Braverman IM, Rousseau ME, Sarrel PM. Skin changes in menopause. Maturitas. 1989;11: 295–304.

49. Varila E, Rantala I, Oikarinen A, Risteli J, Reunala T, Oksanen H, et al. The effect of topical oestradiol on skin collagen of postmenopausal women. Br J Obstet Gynaecol. 1995;102:985–9.

50. Punnonen R, Vaajalahti P, Teisala K. Local oestriol treatment improves the structure of elastic fibers in the skin of postmenopausal women. Ann Chir Gynaecol Suppl. 1987;202:39–41.

51. Henry F, Piérard-Franchimont C, Cauwenbergh G, Piérard GE. Age-related changes in facial skin contours and rheology. J Am Geriatr Soc. 1997;45: 220–2.

52. Piérard GE, Letawe C, Dowlati A, Piérard-Franchimont C. Effect of hormone replacement therapy for menopause on the mechanical properties of skin. J Am Geriatr Soc. 1995;43:662–5.

53. Yoon H-S, Lee S-R, Chung JH. Long-term topical oestrogen treatment of sun-exposed facial skin in post-menopausal women does not improve facial wrinkles or skin elasticity, but induces matrix metalloproteinase-1 expression. Acta Derm Venereol. 2014; 94:4–8.

54. Thornton MJ. Estrogens and aging skin. Dermatoendocrinol. 2013;5:264–70.

55. Ashcroft GS, Greenwell-Wild T, Horan MA, Wahl SM, Ferguson MW. Topical estrogen accelerates cutaneous wound healing in aged humans associated with an altered inflammatory response. Am J Pathol. 1999; 155:1137–46.

56. Margolis DJ, Knauss J, Bilker W. Hormone replacement therapy and prevention of pressure ulcers and venous leg ulcers. Lancet. 2002;359:675–7.

57. Ashcroft GS, Dodsworth J, van Boxtel E, Tarnuzzer RW, Horan MA, Schultz GS, et al. Estrogen accelerates cutaneous wound healing associated with an increase in TGF-beta1 levels. Nat Med. 1997;3: 1209–15.

58. Ashcroft GS, Mills SJ, Lei K, Gibbons L, Jeong MJ, Taniguchi M, et al. Estrogen modulates cutaneous wound healing by downregulating macrophage migration inhibitory factor. J Clin Invest. 2003;111: 1309–18.

59. Nelson HD, Humphrey LL, Nygren P, Teutsch SM, Allan JD. Postmenopausal hormone replacement therapy: scientific review. JAMA. 2002;288:872–81.

60. Warren MP. A comparative review of the risks and benefits of hormone replacement therapy regimens. Am J Obstet Gynecol. 2004;190:1141–67.

61. Surazynski A, Jarzabek K, Haczynski J, Laudanski P, Palka J, Wolczynski S. Differential effects of estradiol and raloxifene on collagen biosynthesis in cultured human skin fibroblasts. Int J Mol Med. 2003;12: 803–9.

62. Sumino H, Ichikawa S, Kasama S, Gibbons L, Jeong MJ, Taniguchi M, et al. Effects of raloxifene and hormone replacement therapy on forearm skin elasticity in postmenopausal women. Maturitas. 2009;62:53–7.

63. Farage MA, Miller KW, Elsner P, Maibach HI. Characteristics of the aging skin. Adv Wound Care. 2013;2:5–10.

64. Yeap BB. Testosterone and ill-health in aging men. Nat Clin Pract Endocrinol Metab. 2009;5:113–21.

65. Sator PG, Schmidt JB, Sator MO, Huber JC, Hönigsmann H. The influence of hormone replacement therapy on skin ageing: a pilot study. Maturitas. 2001;39:43–55.

66. Wright ET, McGillis TJ, Sobel H. Action of testosterone on the skin of aging male subjects. Dermatology. 1970;140:124–8.

67. Brawer MK. Testosterone replacement in men with andropause: an overview. Rev Urol. 2004;6:S9–15.

68. Glaser RL, Dimitrakakis C, Messenger AG. Improvement in scalp hair growth in androgen-deficient women treated with testosterone: a questionnaire study. Br J Dermatol. 2012;166:274–8.

69. Ellis JA, Stebbing M, Harrap SB. Polymorphism of the androgen receptor gene is associated with male pattern baldness. J Invest Dermatol. 2001;116:452–5.

70. Zhuo FL, Xu W, Wang L, Wu Y, Xu ZL, Zhao JY. Androgen receptor gene polymorphisms and risk for androgenetic alopecia: a meta-analysis. Clin Exp Dermatol. 2012;37:104–11.

71. Korting HC, Unholzer A, Schäfer-Korting M, Tausch I, Gassmueller J, Nietsch KH. Different skin thinning potential of equipotent medium-strength glucocorticoids. Skin Pharmacol Appl Skin Physiol. 2002;15: 85–91.

72. Sadagurski M, Yakar S, Weingarten G, Holzenberger M, Rhodes CJ, Breitkreutz D, et al. Insulin-like growth factor 1 receptor signaling regulates skin development and inhibits skin keratinocyte differentiation. Mol Cell Biol. 2006;26:2675–87.

73. Kimura T, Doi K. Dorsal skin reactions of hairless dogs to topical treatment with corticosteroids. Toxicol Pathol. 1999;27:528–35.

74. Lavker RM. Structural alterations in exposed and unexposed aged skin. J Invest Dermatol. 1979; 73:59–66.

75. Lee B, Vouthounis C, Stojadinovic O, Brem H, Im M, Tomic-Canic M. From an enhanceosome to a repressosome: molecular antagonism between glucocorticoids and EGF leads to inhibition of wound healing. J Mol Biol. 2005;345:1083–97.

76. Ashcroft GS, Horan MA, Ferguson MW. Aging is associated with reduced deposition of specific

extracellular matrix components, an upregulation of angiogenesis, and an altered inflammatory response in a murine incisional wound healing model. J Invest Dermatol. 1997;108:430–7.

77. Braverman IM, Fonferko E. Studies in cutaneous aging: I. The elastic fiber network. J Invest Dermatol. 1982;78:434–43.

78. Varani J, Dame MK, Rittie L, Fligiel SE, Kang S, Fisher GJ, et al. Decreased collagen production in chronologically aged skin: roles of age-dependent alteration in fibroblast function and defective mechanical stimulation. Am J Pathol. 2006;168:1861–8.

79. Nuutinen P, Riekki R, Parikka M, Salo T, Autio P, Risteli J, et al. Modulation of collagen synthesis and mRNA by continuous and intermittent use of topical hydrocortisone in human skin. Br J Dermatol. 2003;148:39–45.

80. Autio P, Oikarinen A, Melkko J, Risteli J, Risteli L. Systemic glucocorticoids decrease the synthesis of type I and type III collagen in human skin in vivo, whereas isotretinoin treatment has little effect. Br J Dermatol. 1994;131:660–3.

81. Tiganescu A, Tahrani AA, Morgan SA, Otranto M, Desmoulière A, Abrahams L, et al. 11β-Hydroxysteroid dehydrogenase blockade prevents age-induced skin structure and function defects. J Clin Invest. 2013; 123:3051–60.

82. Tiganescu A, Walker EA, Hardy RS, Mayes AE, Stewart PM. Localization, age- and site-dependent expression, and regulation of 11β-hydroxysteroid dehydrogenase type 1 in skin. J Invest Dermatol. 2011;131:30–6.

83. Chang ALS, Bitter Jr PH, Qu K, Lin M, Rapicavoli NA, Chang HY. Rejuvenation of gene expression pattern of aged human skin by broadband light treatment: a pilot study. J Invest Dermatol. 2013;133:394–402.

84. Apfeld J, Kenyon C. Cell nonautonomy of C. elegans daf-2 Function in the regulation of diapause and life span. Cell. 1998;95:199–210.

85. Kenyon CJ. The genetics of ageing. Nature. 2010; 464:504–12.

86. Suh Y, Atzmon G, Cho MO, Hwang D, Liu B, Leahy DJ, et al. Functionally significant insulin-like growth factor I receptor mutations in centenarians. Proc Natl Acad Sci U S A. 2008;105:3438–42.

87. Vitale G, Brugts MP, Ogliari G, Castaldi D, Fatti LM, Varewijck AJ, et al. Low circulating IGF-I bioactivity is associated with human longevity: findings in centenarians' offspring. Aging. 2012;4:580–9.

88. Sugiyama-Nakagiri Y, Naoe A, Ohuchi A, Kitahara T. Serum levels of IGF-1 are related to human skin characteristics including the conspicuousness of facial pores. Int J Cosmet Sci. 2011;33:144–9.

89. Chang ALS, Atzmon G, Bergman A, Brugmann S, Atwood SX, Chang HY, et al. Identification of genes promoting skin youthfulness by genome-wide association study. J Invest Dermatol. 2014;134:651–7.

90. Sadighi Akha AA, Harper JM, Salmon AB, Schroeder BA, Tyra HM, Rutkowski DT, et al. Heightened induction of proapoptotic signals in response to endoplasmic reticulum stress in primary fibroblasts from a mouse model of longevity. J Biol Chem. 2011;286: 30344–51.

91. Le Clerc S, Taing L, Ezzedine K, Latreille J, Delaneau O, Labib T, et al. A genome-wide association study in Caucasian women points out a putative role of the STXBP5L gene in facial photoaging. J Invest Dermatol. 2013;133:929–35.

92. Tang X, Wang Y, Li D, Luo J, Liu M. Orphan G protein-coupled receptors (GPCRs): biological functions and potential drug targets. Acta Pharmacol Sin. 2012;33:363–71.

Psoriasis Therapy in the Geriatric Population

Daniel C. Butler and John Y.M. Koo

Introduction

The geriatric population of the USA is rapidly growing, and estimates indicate that it will comprise one-fourth of the total population by year 2025 [1]. Such an increase will undoubtedly contribute to an increased prevalence of geriatric patients with psoriasis. One study in the USA showed that the 60–69-year-old age group is most vulnerable to psoriasis [2]. Thus, treating clinicians should be aware of special considerations in treating geriatric psoriasis patients. Physiologic changes associated with aging, concurrent comorbidities, and polypharmacy can all complicate a clinician's treatment approach and lead to inadequate management or undertreatment [3]. However, there are many safe and effective options for older psoriasis patients.

D.C. Butler, M.D. (✉)
Department of Dermatology, Massachusetts General Hospital, 55 Fruit Street, Boston, MA 02114, USA
e-mail: dcbutler@email.arizona.edu

J.Y.M. Koo, M.D.
Professor, Department of Dermatology, UCSF,
515 Spruce Street, San Francisco, CA 94118, USA

Psoriasis Comorbidities in Older Patients

Multiple studies suggest that both mild and severe psoriasis increases the risk of cardiovascular disease, such as myocardial infarction and stroke [4, 5]. The relative risk of cardiovascular death for 60-year-olds with severe psoriasis was estimated at 1.92 (1.41–2.62) [4]. A recent review of literature from the Medical Board of the National Psoriasis Foundation suggests that some psoriasis therapies can decrease cardiovascular disease. Treatments found to decrease cardiovascular risk include methotrexate, tumor necrosis factor inhibitors, and long-term use of ustekinumab [6].

Recently, older psoriatics were found to be more likely to have nonalcoholic fatty liver disease (NAFLD), independent of covariates in both a retrospective and cross-sectional study [7]. The presence of NAFLD should alert physicians to potential liver toxicity with particular treatments for psoriasis such as methotrexate or acitretin, warranting either close monitoring during treatment or avoidance of these hepatotoxic drugs altogether. In addition, NAFLD is associated with metabolic syndrome and is an independent predictor of cardiovascular disease.

Topical Steroids

Topical corticosteroids are the first-line and likely the safest option to treat psoriasis patients. However, the use of topical steroids in geriatric patients poses additional concerns. The risks of increased skin fragility, atrophy, purpura, steroid rebound, skin infections, and telangiectasias are apparent in all ages, but these risks are pronounced in older patients because of the physiologic changes of aging skin [8–10]. Therefore, while the use of topical steroids is recommended as the first-line treatment for elderly individuals by the National Psoriasis Foundation, topical steroids should be prescribed with caution, and clinicians should consider following up with their patients at least once every 3 months to monitor for atrophy [11].

Problems with compliance can further complicate the prescription of topical steroids in the geriatric population. Time and difficulty of application must be considered in light of a patient's physical limitations; patients may struggle with regular use. Prior to prescribing, clinicians should therefore ensure that patients are capable of applying topical agents or be able to receive necessary assistance. Back applicators available from drug stores can help with difficult-to-reach areas such as the back. Combined topical agents may reduce the steps needed for application of two separate drugs in patients with musculoskeletal difficulties. One proven option is combined calcipotriol and betamethasone dipropionate, which is applied once a day and has been proven safe and effective, especially in elderly patients [12].

Phototherapy

Phototherapy is safe and recommended for geriatric patients, although its ability to decrease cardiovascular risk is unproven. Important considerations include the patient's ability to travel to a phototherapy center three times per week as well as physical limitations which may make standing in a phototherapy booth difficult [11].

For instance, older patients in wheelchairs may not be able to stand for the duration of treatment and transportation as well as coordination with caregivers is critical for effective treatment. Narrowband ultraviolet B radiation can be a good choice for older patients with moderate to severe psoriasis if they are able to tolerate positioning in the photo-booth.

Prior to an initial phototherapy session, as well as in subsequent visits, clinicians should conduct a thorough review of the patients' medication list to evaluate for any potentially photosensitizing agent [11, 13]. Phototherapy staff should be reminded to review this list before treatment, paying special attention to any new medications. Phototherapy can be a good choice for patients wishing to avoid drug interaction from concomitant medications.

Traditional Systemics

Response to internal medication can be quite variable in geriatric patients because age-dependent changes in normal physiology alter responses, reactions, and metabolism: organs gradually lose functional capacity, homeostatic mechanisms become slow, fat content increases, and water volume decreases [14]. For traditional systemics, the general rule is to start at a low dose and titrate slowly on the basis of the therapeutic response. Frequent follow-up is recommended to assess adverse effects and degrees of response.

Methotrexate

Methotrexate can be used safely in elderly patients, but the predominant concern is its use with concurrent age-related impaired renal function. Creatinine clearance decreases with age and thus may lead to increased serum concentrations of the medication if dosing is not adjusted by kidney function [15]. For this reason, methotrexate should be initiated at a lower dose than that used for younger psoriasis patients [16]. In addition, elderly patients on methotrexate should be reminded to stay well hydrated. Since these patients have an increased risk of dehydration, methotrexate blood levels may increase to toxic levels.

An additional concern with using methotrexate is the potential for life-threatening myelosuppression. Elderly individuals are often myelosuppressed at baseline, putting them at great risk for these rare but serious adverse events [17]. Typically, a 5 mg "test" dose of methotrexate is given before regular dosing is started. Laboratory evaluations including liver function testing and blood counts are performed before and after the test dose.

Methotrexate can interact with a variety of medications. The most dangerous of these interactions is with the antibiotic trimethoprim, which can result in a fatal reaction [18]. A thorough evaluation of potential interactions with concurrent medications is required for any patient who is starting on a treatment regimen.

Acitretin

Acitretin is the only internal medication that does not have immunosuppressive qualities and is thus appropriate for the geriatric population, although its ability to reduce the rate of cardiovascular events remains to be demonstrated. Additionally, oral retinoids may discourage neoplasm by enhancing cell maturation and differentiation [19]. Their tendency to elevate both triglycerides and cholesterol can be dangerous for patients at risk for coronary disease. The development of hypertriglyceridemia secondary to acitretin use often takes years to develop, so the short-term use of acitretin is likely safe in the geriatric population. While not life threatening, the skin drying effects of acitretin can be particularly concerning in elderly patients who already have a tendency to develop xerosis [11]. The experience of an author (J.K.) has been that low-dose acitretin (10–25 mg/day) is more effective in the geriatric psoriasis patients as compared to younger patients. However, it still takes months to realize this more complete clearing on low-dose acitretin in the elderly.

Cyclosporine

As with the young population, the main concern of using cyclosporine in the elderly population is hypertension and nephrotoxicity [20]. Given that elderly patients have less renal and cardiac reserve, these side effects may be less tolerated. Thus, cyclosporine use in geriatric patients should be limited to the most severe, recalcitrant cases [11]. Trough levels are recommended in the geriatric subgroup if the medication is used in the long term at greater than 3 mg/kg daily; the medication is contraindicated in any patient with an abnormal baseline glomerular filtration rate [21].

Biologics

Because biologic medications are immune-modulating proteins, they are less likely to have the end-organ effects and drug-drug interactions of traditional systemic medications. Moreover, these medications are dosed less frequently than the oral systemic therapies, which can help compliance. The concern is that as individuals age, so does their immune system. Biologics that conferred therapeutic immunosuppression in younger patients may become pathologic in the elderly. With age-related gradual deterioration of the immune system, immunosenescence, and the addition of an immune-suppressing medication, there is a theoretical concern for higher rates of infection and malignancy, but studies on this topic are lacking. The US Food and Drug Administration package inserts for infliximab, ustekinumab, and etanercept do not report any safety issues specific to the geriatric population [22–24]. However, some practitioners avoid using ustekinumab in patients with heart disease due to a controversial and unproven concern for increased cardiovascular risk [25]. Only the FDA package insert of adalimumab warns against a high incidence of serious infections and malignancies in elderly patients [26].

Specific studies on adalimumab and etanercept detail their safe and effective use in elderly patients [27–29]. One study that examined etanercept in a cohort of over 4,000 patients with rheumatoid arthritis, psoriatic arthritis, and ankylosing spondylitis failed to find a higher incidence of serious adverse effects, infectious events, or malignancies in persons over 65 years old compared with those under 65 years of age [30]. Conversely, a different cohort of over 3,000 patients from the British Biologics registry found an increased risk of serious infection for geriatric patients who are taking biologics [31]. While a definitive answer on the absolute safety of biologics remains unclear, biologics can be recommended to elderly patients as long as appropriate caution is taken regarding screening and follow-up.

Recent Studies Comparing Effectiveness and Safety of Psoriasis Treatments in Older Psoriatic Patients

A recent retrospective study of 187 psoriatic patients aged >65 years in Italy examined traditional and biologic treatments and found that biologics (etanercept, adalimumab, infliximab, efalizumab, and ustekinumab) were more effective than traditional treatments (methotrexate, acitretin, cyclosporine, or PUVA) [32]. Etanercept was associated with lowest rate of adverse events per patient-year treated. In the long term, etanercept has lowered cardiovascular risk as well [6].

While the most appropriate treatment for an older psoriatic depends on comorbidities and practical considerations for administration and safety monitoring, future studies should continue to better inform the physician and patient on issues relevant to the geriatric population.

References

1. Bureau UC. Projected resident population of the United States as of July 1, 2025, middle series. Washington, DC: Population Division; 2002.
2. Bell LM, Sedlack R, Beard CM, Perry HO, Michet CJ, Kurland LT. Incidence of psoriasis in Rochester, Minn, 1980–1983. Arch Dermatol. 1991;127(8):1184–7.
3. Wong JW, Koo JY. The safety of systemic treatments that can be used for geriatric psoriasis patients: a review. Dermatol Res Pract. 2012;2012:367475.
4. Mehta NN, Yu Y, Pinnelas R, et al. Attributable risk estimate of severe psoriasis on major cardiovascular events. Am J Med. 2011;124(8):775.e1–6.
5. Armstrong EJ, Harskamp CT, Armstrong AW. Psoriasis and major adverse cardiovascular events: a systematic review and meta-analysis of observational studies. J Am Heart Assoc. 2013;2(2), e000062.
6. Hugh J, Van Voorhees AS, Nijhawan RI, et al. From the Medical Board of the National Psoriasis Foundation: The risk of cardiovascular disease in individuals with psoriasis and the potential impact of current therapies. J Am Acad Dermatol. 2014;70(1):168–77.
7. van der Voort EA, Koehler EM, Dowlatshahi EA, et al. Psoriasis is independently associated with non-alcoholic fatty liver disease in patients 55 years old or older: Results from a population-based study. J Am Acad Dermatol. 2014;70(3):517–24.
8. Coskey RJ. Adverse effects of corticosteroids: I. Topical and intralesional. Clin Dermatol. 1986;4(1): 155–60.
9. du Vivier A, Stoughton RB. Tachyphylaxis to the action of topically applied corticosteroids. Arch Dermatol. 1975;111(5):581–3.
10. Singh G, Singh PK. Tachyphylaxis to topical steroid measured by histamine-induced wheal suppression. Int J Dermatol. 1986;25(5):324–6.
11. Grozdev IS, Van Voorhees AS, Gottlieb AB, et al. Psoriasis in the elderly: from the Medical Board of the National Psoriasis Foundation. J Am Acad Dermatol. 2011;65(3):537–45.
12. Parslew R, Traulsen J. Efficacy and local safety of a calcipotriol/betamethasone dipropionate ointment in elderly patients with psoriasis vulgaris. Eur J Dermatol. 2005;15(1):37–9.
13. Gould JW, Mercurio MG, Elmets CA. Cutaneous photosensitivity diseases induced by exogenous agents. J Am Acad Dermatol. 1995;33(4):551–73. quiz 574-556.
14. Bressler R, Bahl JJ. Principles of drug therapy for the elderly patient. Mayo Clin Proc. 2003;78(12):1564–77.
15. Turnheim K. Drug dosage in the elderly. Is it rational? Drugs Aging. 1998;13(5):357–79.
16. Flammiger A, Maibach H. Drug dosage in the elderly: dermatological drugs. Drugs Aging. 2006;23(3): 203–15.
17. Boffa MJ. Methotrexate for psoriasis: current European practice. A postal survey. J Eur Acad Dermatol Venereol. 2005;19(2):196–202.
18. Evans WE, Christensen ML. Drug interactions with methotrexate. J Rheumatol Suppl. 1985;12 Suppl 12:15–20.
19. Bhutani T, Koo J. A review of the chemopreventative effects of oral retinoids for internal neoplasms. J Drugs Dermatol. 2011;10(11):1292–8.
20. Falck P, Asberg A, Byberg KT, et al. Reduced elimination of cyclosporine A in elderly (>65 years) kidney transplant recipients. Transplantation. 2008;86(10): 1379–83.
21. Heydendael VM, Spuls PI, Ten Berge IJ, Opmeer BC, Bos JD, de Rie MA. Cyclosporin trough levels: is

monitoring necessary during short-term treatment in psoriasis? A systematic review and clinical data on trough levels. Br J Dermatol. 2002;147(1):122–9.

22. Infliximab. (package Insert). Toronto, Canada 2010.

23. Ustekinumab. (package insert). Horsham, PA 2011.

24. Etanercept. (package insert). Thousand Oaks, CA 1998–2011.

25. Reich K, Langley RG, Lebwohl M, et al. Cardiovascular safety of ustekinumab in patients with moderate to severe psoriasis: results of integrated analyses of data from phase II and III clinical studies. Br J Dermatol. 2011;164(4):862–72.

26. Adalimumab. (package insert). North Chicago, Ill 2002.

27. Gottlieb AB, Boehncke WH, Darif M. Safety and efficacy of alefacept in elderly patients and other special populations. J Drugs Dermatol. 2005;4(6):718–24.

28. Militello G, Xia A, Stevens SR, Van Voorhees AS. Etanercept for the treatment of psoriasis in the elderly. J Am Acad Dermatol. 2006;55(3):517–9.

29. Menter A, Gordon KB, Leonardi CL, Gu Y, Goldblum OM. Efficacy and safety of adalimumab across subgroups of patients with moderate to severe psoriasis. J Am Acad Dermatol. 2010;63(3):448–56.

30. Fleischmann R, Baumgartner SW, Weisman MH, Liu T, White B, Peloso P. Long term safety of etanercept in elderly subjects with rheumatic diseases. Ann Rheum Dis. 2006;65(3):379–84.

31. Galloway JB, Hyrich KL, Mercer LK, et al. Anti-TNF therapy is associated with an increased risk of serious infections in patients with rheumatoid arthritis especially in the first 6 months of treatment: updated results from the British Society for Rheumatology Biologics Register with special emphasis on risks in the elderly. Rheumatology (Oxford). 2011;50(1):124–31.

32. Piaserico S, Conti A, Lo Console F, et al. Efficacy and safety of systemic treatments for psoriasis in elderly patients. Acta Derm Venereol. 2014;94(3):293–7.

Supportive Skin Care in Older Patients

Staci Brandt and Matthew Meckfessel

Supportive skin care as described in this chapter includes skin care regimens that promote and maintain healthy skin barrier in older patients. It may be used with or without prescribed medications or treatments.

According to the United Nation's World Population Ageing Report published in 2007, population aging is reaching unprecedented levels, and having a profound implication worldwide for all facets of human life [1]. In 2000, the number of people in the world aged 60 years or over numbered 600 million. By 2050, this number is projected to grow to over two billion [1]. This pervasive change in population requires healthcare workers to better understand the medical needs of this growing demographic.

As the proportion of the US senior population continues to increase so does the number of outpatient visits to both general practitioners and specialists, including dermatologists [2]. It is estimated that 7 % of all physician visits by the elderly involve skin disorders, and that treatable, but often untreated, cutaneous diseases occur in greater than 50 % of otherwise healthy adults [2]. Effective management of these dermatology conditions requires healthcare providers to be prepared to monitor cutaneous health in aging patients and recognize signs of impending cutaneous breakdown [3]. Foundational knowledge in the physiologic and morphologic changes, clinical considerations, and effective management and supportive skin care options for older patients will lead to more optimal patient outcomes in this growing population.

Physiologic and Morphologic Cutaneous Changes in Older Skin

As with many other organ systems, the skin suffers progressive morphologic and physiologic decrements with time, though the fundamental pathophysiologic mechanisms involved in aging skin are still under study [1]. There is a growing body of evidence indicating that these pathophysiologic mechanisms are multifactorial [3–6]. The research in aging skin has shown that changes of skin aging are a consequence of damage caused by both intrinsic (physiological mechanisms and genetic predisposition) and extrinsic factors (external insults, particularly solar radiation) [7].

A minority of research in skin aging focuses on the mechanisms of skin barrier differences, both intrinsic and extrinsic. However, there are data suggesting that epidermal function can be

S. Brandt, PA-C, M.B.A., M.S. (✉)
Corporate Medical Affairs, Galderma Spirig,
Egerkingen, Switzerland
e-mail: staci.brandt@galderma.com

M. Meckfessel, Ph.D.
Medical Communications, 14501N Freeway,
Fort Worth, TX 76244, USA
e-mail: matthew.meckfessel@galderma.com

© Springer International Publishing Switzerland 2015
A.L.S. Chang (ed.), *Advances in Geriatric Dermatology*, DOI 10.1007/978-3-319-18380-0_6

altered by controlling the balance of water and ions in the body [7]. Additional insights into the literature include studies that show that filaggrin is immunohistochemically decreased in aged skin when compared to levels in young skin [5]. Total ceramide content in the stratum corneum significantly declines with age [5, 6]. Free amino acid content of natural moisturizing factor and aquaporin 3 (AQP3) expression have also been reported to be lower in aging epidermis [7].

Age-related changes in the stratum corneum include reduced water content, decreased number of lipids, increased number and size of corneocytes, decreased size of sebaceous gland, decreased size of sweat glands, and reduced vasculature [2]. Lipid synthesis and secretion of lamellar bodies in the stratum corneum diminish with age, which causes a more porous extracellular matrix and less efficient water-ion balance [7]. All of these pathophysiologic states can lead to impaired barrier function that becomes progressively more compromised [3].

Additionally the loss of collagen and elastin fibers in the dermis can reduce the tensile strength of the skin, and progressive vasculature atrophies can leave patients more susceptible to status dermatitis, pressure ulcers, and skin tears [3]. Lastly, the cumulative effects of environmental insults, particularly exposure to solar radiation, also contribute to the marked increase in neoplastic disease [4].

All of these findings indicate that aging skin undergoes a progressive degenerative change and that the consequences of both intrinsic and extrinsic influences may result in a marked susceptibility to dermatologic disorders in the elderly [8].

Clinical Considerations in Aging Skin

Molecular and cell-related changes in the ageing epidermis also contribute to the clinical presentation of dermatologic conditions. Xerosis and pruritus are the most commonly observed signs and symptoms in elderly patients [8]. Other clinical presentations related to stratum corneum include increased predisposition to formation or deepening wrinkles, fragility and difficulty to heal injuries, alteration in skin permeability to drugs, impaired ability to sense and respond to mechanical stimuli, and skin irritation [7].

While elderly patients can present with a myriad of dermatologic disorders, xerosis has been reported as a common condition in this population. The prevalence of xerosis has been reported to be up to 38.9 % and also reference other studies reporting prevalence ranging from 29.5 to 58.3 % [2]. Xerosis typically presents as dry, rough, scaling skin [2]. Xerosis results from a disruption in the complex balance of normal hydration and results in markedly higher transepidermal water loss (TEWL) and lower skin surface hydration [9]. Additionally, abnormal permeability barrier in aged skin suggests that the basis for the defect is a result of a delay in lipid processing and a defective acidification of the stratum corneum. This abnormal stratum corneum acidification could be responsible for the multiple defects seen in epidermal function including delayed permeability barrier recovery after external perturbation and abnormal stratum corneum integrity [10]. Corneocytes can desquamate in clumps of cell aggregates and the stratum corneum can become thicker and dryer [9]. Patients xerois has been cited as the most common cause of pruritus in older adults [2]. Complications from pruritus include skin excoriations, secondary infections, disruption in sleep patterns, and in some patients the development of chronic wounds [2]. Effective therapy for pruritus can be challenging and suggest an individually tailored approach with consideration for a patient's general health, severity of symptoms, and adverse events of available treatments [8]. While there are topical and systemic treatments available for pruritus, it is important to remember that the physical and cognitive limitations such as impaired vision, hearing, and mobility are not uncommon in this population [3].

Additionally, multiple comorbid conditions and polypharmacy of this age group are critical variables to consider when making a treatment decision [8]. Data has shown that 13 % of the US population is over the age of 65 years and this demographic utilizes one-third of all prescription medicines [11]. Prevalence of polypharmacy substantially increases the risk of cutaneous drug reactions, many of which include pruritus as a symptom [3]. A case–control study reported that calcium channel blockers were associated with chronic eczematous eruptions in the elderly subjects with symptoms of itching [12]. Anecdotally, cooling topical agents such as Sarna lotion, calamine, or zinc oxide paste may at least temporarily ameliorate the symptoms of itching.

Another comorbid condition that associates with the older population is incontinence. Either urinary or fecal incontinence may lead to moisture and maceration in the skin folds. This exposure then causes intertrigo, irritant contact dermatitis, or fungal and bacterial infections. Supportive skin care is critical to avoiding these conditions. These minimize time of exposure to urine or feces with frequent diaper changes, use of highly absorbant adult diapers, skin barrier creams such as zinc oxide, and avoidance of paper wipes that may contain chemical associated with contact allergy [13]. More recently, split body studies of intertrigo have demonstrated equal efficacy of honey barrier cream and zinc oxide ointment for intertrigo with the honey barrier cream showing less pruritus complaints [14].

Significant Impact on Quality of Life

Cutaneous diseases carry with them significant morbidity and the potential to greatly decrease the patient's quality of life [3]. Data examining psychological implications of dermatologic conditions in the aging population, including severe xerosis, highlighted that people tend to resist intimate contact with the elderly, causing the elderly to feel rejected with less motivation to take care of themselves [15]. Whatever makes an older person appear less attractive can have an unfavorable effect upon opportunities to make use of society's life support systems [15].

Management of Aging Skin and Supportive Skin Care

Effective management of dermatologic conditions in aging skin conditions requires distinguishing between lesions that are a normal part of aging and those which are clinically significant, which should be treated and may be a sign of impending cutaneous breakdown [3]. Treatment plans may be modified to meet the needs of the elderly patient, and take into consideration their increased skin fragility, numerous comorbidities, probable polypharmacy, and possible lack of mobility and social support [3]. Appropriate care, continuing surveillance by practitioners of their patients' skin, judicious limitation of unnecessary risk factors (particularly exposure to solar radiation), and prompt, relevant, and thoughtful treatment of any clinically significant cutaneous disorder can prolong life and substantially improve the quality of life of patients during their later years [3].

The keys to xerosis management include restoration of the damaged stratum corneum barrier and maintenance of the moisture content [2]. Xerosis is most commonly treated with topically applied moisturizers [16]. Moisturizers alleviate dry skin and primary irritation and can prevent symptoms associated with xerosis [17]. Moisturizers may be formulated with many ingredients, with humectants and emollients being two important classes of ingredients [18]. Humectants increase hydration by drawing moisture through the stratum corneum. Emollients are lipid-based ingredients that can make the skin soft and pliable by increasing hydration and also help maintain barrier integrity [18]. Additionally, occlusive ingredients such as petrolatum can provide a barrier on the surface of the skin to slow water loss and thus increase the moisture content of the stratum corneum [19].

Despite the numerous moisturizers available to consumers, xerosis and pruritus continue to remain significant problems for elderly patients. Some moisturizers are formulated with ingredients that maintain and improve barrier function, while other ingredients may actually be detrimental

Table 1 Common ingredients in skin care products

Substance	Component of the skin	Can be found in moisturizers	Substance	Component of the skin	Can be found in moisturizers
Glycerol	X	X	Tocopherol	X	X
Triglycerides	X	X	Almond oil		X
Petrolatum		X	Lactic acid	X	X
Dexpanthenol	X	X	Lanolin		X
Urea	X	X	Phytosterols	X	X
Salicylic acid		X	Evening prime rose oil		X
Ceramides	X	X	Fatty acids/essential fatty acids	X	X
Zinc		X	Cholesterol	X	X
Silver		X	Squalene/squalane		X
Aluminum		X	Vitamin B_3	X	X

to the stratum corneum [16]. Table 1 outlines ingredients commonly used in skin care products available to support barrier function:

Glycerol is a trivalent alcohol that dissolves well in water. It is the backbone of triglycerides and is a component in natural moisturizing factor in the stratum corneum. Glycerol provides barrier-stabilizing properties through intensive hydration of the stratum corneum [20].

Triglycerides are chemical compounds built of three molecules of fatty acid combined with one molecule of glycerol. They are the source of fatty acids for skin metabolism and are a major component of the lipid barrier of the stratum corneum.

Petrolatum is the first known barrier product and is the gold standard among barrier repair ingredients. It is the closest ingredient to natural intercellular lipids and is widely used as an emollient and vehicle in cosmetics and personal care products. Petrolatum helps slow water loss from the skin by forming an occlusive barrier on the skin's surface [21].

Dexpanthenol (vitamin B5) is a stable alcoholic analog of pantothenic acid that serves as an essential compound in skin metabolism and normal epithelial function. Dexpanthenol improves stratum corneum hydration, reduces transepidermal water loss, and helps maintain skin softness and elasticity. It has also been shown to significantly accelerate epidermal regeneration and is well tolerated [22].

Table 2 Intracellular matrix composition

Lipids	Percentage in the SC^a (%)
Ceramide	50
Cholesterol	35
Long-chain free fatty acid	10–20

Adapted from [23] Sugarman, J. The Epidermal Barrier in Atopic Dermatitits. Semin Cutan Med Surg 27:108–114, 2008
[a]Percentages are approximate estimates

Cholesterol, ceramides, and fatty acids are lipids that help form the permeability barrier of the skin and are major components of the intercellular matrix in the stratum corneum (Table 2). They are important for reducing TEWL and essential for normal permeability barrier function [23].

Phytosterols are sterols from plants (e.g., shea butter) and soothe skin by reducing inflammatory mediators (prostaglandins and leukotrienes). They help to reinforce the skin barrier and can be helpful in inflammatory skin disease (e.g., atopic dermatitis) [24].

Squalene/squalane is a natural organic compound and natural moisturizer related to skin lipids.

Vitamin B_3 (niacinamide) is a water-soluble vitamin that helps the stimulation of the biosynthesis of natural ceramides and intracellular lipids. It has anti-inflammatory effects, reduces TEWL, and improves skin barrier function. Niacinamide has also been demonstrated to have a smoothing effect or improvement in the skin surface [25].

In vitro data has shown niacinamide to stimulate collagen synthesis and to up-regulate epidermal sphingolipids, particularly ceramides [16].

Tocopherol (vitamin E) is used in concentrations 2–20 % and has been known to soothe the skin, increase moisture levels in the stratum corneum, and accelerate the epithelialization of the skin [25], although low rates of allergic contact dermatitis have been reported [26].

Lanolin is a yellow waxy substance secreted by the sebaceous glands of wool-bearing animals. Lanolin is a natural protection for skin against environmental influences and contains no triglycerides (unlike human sebum) [27]. Jennings et al. have shown that pure lanolin and ammonium lactate 12 % cream are both effective in treating xerosis when used twice daily for 4 weeks [28]. Furthermore, ammonium lactate can reduce the pH of stratum corneum promoting dissociation of overly retained corneocytes and thinning out hyperkeratotic skin.

Lactic acid is another strong humectant with moisture-retaining properties. Lactic acid is also a keratolytic ingredient [29]. Lactic acid functions as a modulator of skin keratinization by producing epidermal proliferation, which creates a stimulatory response [9]. Lactic acid has also been identified as a pH adjuster and a mild exfoliant [9, 30].

Urea is a humectant frequently used in dermatology [9]. Urea has been shown to hydrate the SC (hygroscopic effect), reduce TEWL, improve skin barrier function, and soothe pruritus. Urea has keratolytic properties and is a component of natural moisturizing factor [31]. Urea is a nontoxic ingredient that can elicit concentration-dependent desquamating effects on the stratum corneum [9].

While moisturizers can help treat xerosis by replacing water content and maintaining hydration, alleviating symptomatology, and controlling keratinization, therapy should not be limited to only topical application of moisturizers. Bathing routines should include the use of a mild moisturizing soap or soap substitute that doesn't irritate the skin [2]. Avoid cleansers with a high pH or those containing alcohol, in addition to using moisturizers or barrier creams regularly (ideally with a low pH) [8].

There are a number of general measures that may be useful in managing pruritus in the elderly irrespective of the underlying cause such as patient education, identifying and removing the aggravating factors, and breaking the "itch-scratch" cycle which causes increased cutaneous inflammation [8]. Patel et al. also suggest simple measures such as keeping the finger nails short, tepid showering, wearing light clothing, and using air conditioning to keep skin cool, which can also help support the pruritus found in aging skin [8].

Clinical Pearls in Supportive Skin Care in Older Patients

In dermatology clinic, older patients with xerosis are counseled on skin care regimens that minimize loss of skin barrier components. While these are not systematically studies, they comprise practical suggestions from clinical experience. These include keeping baths and showers short (less than 5 min), using lukewarm not hot water, minimizing exposures to soap and detergent, and applying a thick cream moisturizer after bathing [8]. Minimizing exposures to soap and detergents include applying them only to the scalp, axillae, groin, and feet. Other body areas do not need soap unless visibly soiled. Compared to traditional soaps, syndets typically have a lower pH, which is less irritating and less disruptive to skin barrier function [10]. However, some syndets may have an alkaline pH, often higher than traditional soaps, and be just as irritating. Many products are also blends of soap and syndet and clinicians should be aware of these differences and their potential for irritation when making product recommendations.

References

1. UN Aging Report- http://www.un.org/esa/population/publications/publications.htm
2. White-Chu E, Reddy M. Dry skin in elderly: complexities of a common problem. Clin Dermatol. 2011; 29:37–42.
3. Farage MA, Miller KW, Berardesca E, Maibach HI. Clinical Implications of aging skin: cutaneous disorders in the elderly. Am J Clin Dermatol. 2009;10(2):73–86.

4. Zouboulis CC, Makrantonaki E. Clinical aspects of molecular diagnostics of skin aging. Clin Dermatol. 2011;29:3–14.

5. Takahashi M, Tezuka T. The content of free amino acids in the stratum corneum is increased in senile xerosis. Arch Dermatol Res. 2004;295:448–52.

6. Imokawa G, Abe A, Jin K, Higaki Y, Kawashima M, Hidano A. Decreased level of ceramides in stratum corneum of atopic dermatitis: an etiologic factor dry skin? J Invest Dermatol. 1991;94(4):523–6.

7. Lorencini M, Brohem CA, Dieamant GC, Zanchin NI, Maibach HI. Active ingredients against human epidermal aging. Ageing Res Rev. 2014;15:100–15. PubMed PMID: 24675046.

8. Patel T, Yosipovitch G. The management of chronic pruritus in the elderly. Skin Therapy Lett. 2010;15(8):5–10.

9. Ademola J, Frazier C, Kim SJ, Theaux C, Saudez X. Clinical evaluation of 40 % urea and 12 % ammonium lactate in the treatment of xerosis. Am J Clin Dermatol. 2002;3(3):217–22. PubMed PMID: 11978141.

10. Baranda L, Gonzalez-Amaro R, Torres-Alvarez B, Alvarez C, Ramírez V. Correlation between pH and irritant effect of cleansers marketed for dry skin. Int J Dermatol. 2002;41:494–9.

11. Joly P, Benoit-Corven C, Baricault S, Lambert A, Hellot MF, Josset V, et al. Chronic eczematous eruptions of the elderly are associated with chronic exposure to calcium channel blockers: results from a case-control study. J Invest Dermatol. 2007;127:2766–71.

12. Schmutz JL, Barbaud A, Tréchot P. Lisinopril-induced erythroderma. Ann Dermatol Vernereol. 2009;136:486.

13. Farage MA, Miller KW, Berardesca E, Maibach HI. Incontinence in the aged: contact dermatitis and other cutaneous consequences. Contact Dermatitis. 2007;57(4):211–7.

14. Nijhuis WA, Houwing RH, Van der Zwet WC, Jansman FG. A randomised trial of honey barrier cream versus zinc oxide ointment. Br J Nursing. 2012;21(20):9–10, 12–3.

15. Kligman A, Koblenzer C. Demographics and psychological implications for the aging population. Dermatol Clin. 1997;15(4):549–53.

16. Christman JC, Fix DK, Lucus SC, Watson D, Desmier E, Wilkerson RJ, et al. Two randomized, controlled, comparative studies of the stratum corneum integrity benefits of two cosmetic niacinamide/glycerin body moisturizers vs. conventional body moisturizers. J Drugs Dermatol. 2012;11(1):22–9. PubMed PMID: 22206073.

17. Simion FA, Abrutyn ES, Draelos ZD. Ability of moisturizers to reduce dry skin and irritation and to prevent their return. Int J Cosmet Sci. 2006;28:232.

18. Bikowski J. The use of therapeutic moisturizers in various dermatologic disorders. Cutis. 2001;68:3–11.

19. Kraft JN, Lynde CW. Moisturizers: what they are and a practical approach to product selection. Skin Therapy Lett. 2005;10.

20. Fluhr JW, Darlenski R, Surber C. Glycerol and the skin: holistic approach to its origin and functions. Br J Dermatol. 2008;159:23–34.

21. Draelos ZD. New treatments for restoring impaired epidermal barrier permeability: Skin barrier repair creams. Clin Dermatol. 2012;30:345–8.

22. Ebner F, Heller A, Rippke F, Tausch I. Topic use of Dexpanthenol in skin disorders. Am J Clin Dermatol. 2002;3:427–33.

23. Sugarman JL. The epidermal barrier in atopic dermatitis. Semin Cutan Med Surg. 2008;27:108–14.

24. Raab VW, Kindl U. Pflegekosmetik—Ein Leitfaden. Stuttgart: Fischer Verlag; 1991.

25. Elsner P, Fluhr JW, Gehring W, Kerscher MJ, Krutmann J, Lademann J, et al. Anti-aging data and support claims—consensus statement. J Dtsch Dermatol Ges. 2001;9 Suppl 3:S1–S32.

26. Kosari P, Alikhan A, Sockolov M, Feldman SR. Vitamin E and allergic contact dermatitis. Dermatitis. 2010;21(3):148–53.

27. Lodén M. Role of topical emollients and moisturizers in the treatment of dry skin barrier disorders. Am J Clin Dermatol. 2003;4:771–88.

28. Jennings MB, Alfieri DM, Parker ER, Jackman L, Goodwin S, Lesczczynski C. A double-blind clinical trial comparing the efficacy and safety of pure lanolin versus ammonium lactate 12 % cream for the treatment of moderate to severe foot xerosis. Cutis. 2003;71(1):78–82. PubMed PMID: 12553635.

29. Raab W, Kindl U. Pflegekosmetik – Ein Leitfaden. 5. Auflage 2012; Wissenschaftliche Verlagsgesellschaft Stuttgart

30. Loden M, von Scheele J, Michelson S. The influence of a humectant rich mixture on normal skin barrier function and on once and twice daily treatment of foot xerosis: a prospective randomized evaluator blind bilateral and untreated control study. Skin Res Tech. 2013;19:438–45.

31. Pan M, Heinecke G, Bernardo S, Tsui C, Levitt J. Urea: a comprehensive review of the clinical literature. Dermatol Online J. 2013;19(11):1. available from http://escholarship.org/uc/item/11x463rp; last accessed May 2014.

Long-Term Care Dermatology

Robert A. Norman

Introduction

The Graying of America

Today, more than 38 million Americans are senior citizens. The number will rise to 53 million by 2020, and 70 million by 2030. The number of those over 65 has increased 100 % between 1960 and 1994. America's 65-and-over population will increase from one in eight to one in five people by 2050. The "oldest old" group, a term describing people over 85, has increased by 274 % during that same time, to more than 3.5 million. The number will likely rise up to 27 million by 2050 if improvements in medical care continue to prolong lives.

Florida has the highest percentage of seniors, with 19 % of its residents 65 and above. The 2012 US Census estimates show that 18.2 % of Floridians are over age 65, the highest rate of any state in the nation.

Read more: http://www.kmbc.com/florida-has-highest-rate-of-seniors/20551672#ixzz3 DLo4due7. By 2020, Florida's share is expected to be 25.6 %.

R.A. Norman (✉)
University of Central Florida, College of Medicine,
8002 Gunn Highway, Tampa, FL 33626, USA
e-mail: skindrrob@aol.com

Needs

Although seniors are better educated, financially solvent, and healthier than ever before, the large increases projected in the elderly population in the next century will increase the strains on medical safety nets. The oldest old are most likely to be poor and prone to multiple chronic diseases and disabilities, and the least likely to have networks of family supports (http://www.ahrq. gov/research/findings/factsheets/aging/elderdis/ index.html).

Legal and Financial Burden

A brief legal overview of patient care in the nursing home includes several items. A do not resuscitate (*DNR*) provides specific instruction to the health care staff pertaining to resuscitation, chest compressions, and mechanical ventilation. A *living will* enables an adult with the capacity to leave written instructions regarding future care in the event the individual is incapable of decision making. A *health care proxy appointment* enables an adult with the capacity to appoint an agent and an alternate agent for health care decisions in case of future incapacity. Individuals entering nursing homes have frequently already lost the capacity to participate in many but not necessarily

A.L.S. Chang (ed.), *Advances in Geriatric Dermatology*, DOI 10.1007/978-3-319-18380-0_7

all medical decisions. In dermatology, the situations we commonly deal with in the nursing home setting include capacity to consent, and quality-of-life issues. Even if a condition is not curable, the patient's quality of life can be significantly improved by reducing pain and itch related to skin.

In 1987 Congress enacted legislation to require nursing homes participating in the Medicare and Medicaid programs to comply with certain requirements for quality of care. Included is the Omnibus Budget Reconciliation Act of 1987 (OBRA 1987), also known as the Nursing Home Reform Act. It specifies that a nursing home "must provide services and activities to attain or maintain the highest practicable physical, mental, and psychosocial well-being of each resident in accordance with a written plan of care ...."

Facilities

Nursing Homes

Nursing homes provide health care, social services, and a homelike environment to people who can no longer live alone and individuals whose care needs exceed the abilities of their families to meet. Nursing homes serve not only the elderly, but also the disabled children and young adults who are chronically ill or have been injured in accidents.

Medical and Administrative Structures of Extended Care Facilities

Ownership

Of the 15,700 nursing homes in the USA, approximately 15,000 are owned by individual or corporate private entrepreneurs and operate the facilities as for-profit business. Approximately 68.2 % of these for-profit homes are owned by chains, and the number is rising. The others are usually family-owned and -managed operations. The largest of the publicly owned and traded chains is the California-based Beverly Enterprises that operates more than 1,000 facilities in 46 states. Washington-based Hillhaven Corporation has close to 400 homes in 40 states. Dallas's

National Heritage and Houston's ARA Living Centers each has more than 200 homes. Manor Care, based in Maryland, and Milwaukee-based Unicare both have more than 100 homes.

Long-term care facilities are often referred to by the level of care they provide. While the federal government has eliminated distinctions between levels of care, referring to all nursing homes as "nursing facilities" and requiring all facilities to meet the same federal standards (http://www. ncdhhs.gov/dma/nursingfacility/ChapterFour. pdf), the standard levels of care are still based on the following:

Level I

Level I facilities are intensive nursing and rehabilitative care facilities which provide continuous skilled nursing care. Many nursing home facilities now have subacute sections, which accommodate patients who have just undergone surgeries or need intensive rehabilitation outside of the hospital setting.

Level II

Level II facilities provide skilled nursing care which is the level of care most closely approximating hospital care. Skilled facilities provide specialized nursing care 24 h a day and rehabilitative services such as physical, occupational, and speech therapy.

Level III

Level III facilities provide intermediate nursing care that consists of routine nursing care 24 h a day and assistance with activities of daily living such as eating, dressing, toileting, and bathing. They also provide rehabilitative services as needed.

Level IV

Level IV facilities are rest homes, which provide protective supervision for individuals who do not routinely require nursing or medical care.

Who Needs Nursing Home Care?

Each year almost 1.5 million people are admitted to the more than 20,000 nursing homes in the USA. The average nursing home resident is a woman in her 80s with three or four chronic illnesses (http://aspe.hhs.gov/daltcp/reports/diseldes.htm). The majority of nursing home residents are admitted from hospitals after experiencing some type of acute medical problem which has impaired their ability to function independently.

Nursing home residents typically have a variety of physical and cognitive disabilities. Close to half are unable to make decisions on their own, and about a third are non-ambulatory. National studies have indicated that up to half of all nursing home residents may have Alzheimer's disease or a related disorder. Some people may remain in a nursing home for only a few months as they recuperate from an illness or operation. Others may require nursing home care for a number of years. The average length of stay is slightly less than 2 years. About 20 % of nursing home residents are able to be discharged to their homes after a period of rehabilitation in a nursing home.

Nursing home and other long-term care needs increase with age. Only about 5 % of those between 65 and 85 need nursing home care, but nearly a quarter of all Americans 85 and older have spent time in a nursing home. Some people may remain in a nursing home for a short time as they recuperate from an illness or operation. The rise of subacute facilities that focus on patients recently discharged from the hospital is growing; many facilities now have a subacute section in their facility. About 20 % of nursing home residents are able to be discharged to their home after a period of rehabilitation in a nursing *home*.

Who Assures the Quality of Care in Nursing Homes?

All nursing homes are inspected at least once a year by the Department of Public Health. State inspectors look at everything from the adequacy of staffing to the cleanliness of the facility to food preparation and the proper administration of medications. In addition, nursing homes are required to meet stringent state and federal fire safety standards.

Most nursing homes have adopted a number of specific laws and programs to further protect the safety and welfare of nursing home residents, including:

A patient's bill of rights

A nursing home receivership law which allows the state to petition the courts for the appointment of an outside receiver to manage facilities where poor patient care is being provided

A patient abuse law which protects nursing home residents from abuse, mistreatment, and neglect by requiring caregivers to report suspected cases of abuse

A nursing home suitability law which requires the Department of Public Health to screen all prospective buyers of nursing homes

A nursing home ombudsman program, which provides volunteer ombudsmen to visit nursing home residents on a weekly basis to resolve any complaints or concerns they may have

Basics of Nursing Home Management

The nursing home administrator, licensed by the state, provides the daily management of a nursing home. The administrator generally has a combination of education in health care administration and experience in the field. Continuing education requirements are necessary for re-licensure.

The administrator has a crucial role in the nursing home. The job consists of translating the federal and state rules and regulations as well as the policies of the owner or governing body into the operations of the home.

All nursing homes have physicians designated as medical directors. Beyond the state mandated minimum, however, there is generally not a significant medical presence in any of the nursing homes. Typically the medical director spends a few hours per week in the home checking on residents and medical orders. In some of the larger institutions, however, there are full-time medical directors. Each resident is required to have an attending physician.

Usually the attending physician is notified by the nursing director or nurse manager that a certain patient requires dermatological evaluation and therapy. In cases when a procedure cannot be done in-house, the patient may be sent out for more extensive treatment.

In many cases, the attending doctor is also the medical director, but the resident has the right to select his or her own physician. A dermatologist who wishes to provide services must apply for privileges to the medical director and nursing home administrator. These privileges can include skin biopsies, cryotherapy, excisions, vaccinations, or mobile superficial radiation units. Consents for treatment if nursing home residents are not able to do so on their own can be arranged through a family member or other legally authorized representative.

Basics of the Nursing Staff

Nursing generally represents 60 % of the total employee complement of any long-term care facility. Registered nurses, licensed practical nurses, and aides are the three distinct groups providing care. The aides typically make up 70 % of the nursing staff. Each generally requires between 80 and 100 h of training before certification. The aides are central to the delivery of daily care, including bathing, dressing, feeding, and transporting the residents. The aides can be critical to identifying lesions and conditions during bathing and dressing especially if the patient has vision or cognitive disabilities. The frequency of physician examinations/visits varies depending on state regulations.

Each resident requires a different amount of nursing time. The crucial measure is "hours of nursing care per resident per day." With the advent of PPS, each home is allotted a certain amount of remuneration based upon the amount of nursing care needed for each patient.

The director of nursing (DON) is generally the physician's primary contact when it comes to nursing home consultations. The DON provides a list of the patients needed to be seen, and acts as a liaison between the nursing home patient and the attending physician, ensuring that the orders are placed and all the specialists are notified. The social service director may also act as the intermediary for consultations. It is important to know who are the key people when it comes to consultations and getting orders carried out within each facility that you may attend.

Many therapeutic services are available in the nursing home including physical, occupational, speech, art, music, and pet therapy. Physical and occupational therapy are two of the primary treatments, which include restoration of function, prevention of disability, and relief of pain. Physical therapists usually develop a treatment plan. It is part of an evaluation that includes test of muscle strength, gait analysis, body part measurements, and a range of motion assessment. Treatments may include whirlpools, ultrasound, hot packs, massage, parallel bars, and a variety of muscle-building devices such as wall pulleys. Occupational therapists concentrate on channeling the strength developed in physical therapy into daily living activities, such as arts and crafts, and homemaking skills. Many facilities have an activity director. Arts and crafts, exercise, current event discussions, games such as bingo, and religious services are some of the activities in which residents participate. In addition, there is often a library for the residents' edification. Often trips are provided to places such as museums or the racetrack.

A consulting dietician is a key part of the nursing home makeup. Often the physician will order a special diet, such as low cholesterol or low fat, and the dietician reviews the diet and insures that it is adequate in all aspects. Significant differences in how meals are planned, prepared, and delivered make for a demanding job.

In addition to the previously mentioned employees, there are many others who are involved with the smooth operation of a good-quality nursing home. Laundry workers deal with the institution's laundry as well as the personal clothing of the residents, maintenance workers insure the mechanical functioning and safety of the facility, and housekeeping staffs keep the facility presentable and inoffensive. Business office people pay bills, order supplies, bill the residents, and may act as personal bankers for residents. The entire group of employees act as a surrogate family for the residents. Their caring attitude and behavior make all the difference between one home and another, between a pleasant and rewarding experience and a degrading experience.

Think about it. What happens if you were in a situation where you are now put into a facility such as a nursing home? The nurses and aides would help you get out of bed in the morning, toilet, bath, dress, eat, and take your medications. The activities' staff would be around you attempting to stimulate your interest and zest for life. The food service personnel would be cooking for your health and enjoyment and therapists would be busy fighting an uphill battle against a possibly deteriorating body and mind, and the social service staff would try to help solve problems ranging from financial difficulties to unpleasant roommates. Although many social service people act as marketing operatives, with the primary function of recruiting residents, most social service directors that I have encountered help educate families about themselves, their needs, and the resources that are available in the community to serve these needs.

As a health care provider, we enter into the resident's home, a place that is often new and sometimes permanent. It is important to keep that in mind. In order to become part of the resident's life and therapeutic family, you must keep a respect for the resident and his/her environment. Many move into nursing homes from their own residents or those of family and friends and the rest are transferred directly from hospitals to nursing homes. The patient and family are under considerable pressure. Very often a long period of adjustment is needed, coming to grips with the fact that many of these residents will never return to their previous homes or lifestyle.

Other Facilities

There are many other ways to accommodate those who need chronic care. The Adult Congregate Living Facility (ACLF) is filled with people who generally do not require as much care as the skilled nursing facilities or what we call nursing homes. In addition, there are many retirement homes, rest homes, and private homes that can provide excellent care for those disabled or those with chronic needs.

Goals of care in an institutional setting may differ from those of the acute hospital. The emphasis is placed on maximizing function, maintaining quality of life, and comfort care rather than curing disease. It is important to communicate with the resident's family, to address their fears and concerns, when present, and to ensure their participation in the development of the care plan. Follow-up care includes interventions to handle acute events, periodic reassessments of the patient's status, and implementation of preventative programs to meet the specific goals of the resident. Scheduled evaluations and sick visits provide an opportunity to review the resident's and staffs' concerns, monitor vital signs including weight, identify changes in the physical examination, reexamine the medication list, and review the care plan.

Advanced Directives

Evaluating nursing home residents about medical decision-making capacity and securing of advance directives are essential to quality care. Advance directives such as the DNR, living will, and health care proxy appointment should be secured as part of the admission assessment. Residents' fears regarding illness and dying should be explored and their wishes regarding resuscitation, hospitalization, and medical interventions should be discussed.

The geriatric long-term care population often suffers from dementia resulting in a progressive cognitive impairment that makes this vulnerable group unable to express their wishes or participate fully in their own care. Advanced directives can facilitate the decision-making process that respects a resident's values and wishes.

A DNR gives specific instruction to the health care staff pertaining to resuscitation, chest compressions, and mechanical ventilation. A living will enables an adult with the capacity to leave written instructions regarding future care in the event the individual is incapable of decision making. A health care proxy appointment enables an adult with the capacity to appoint an agent and an alternate agent for health care decisions in case of future incapacity. Individuals entering nursing homes have frequently already lost the capacity to participate in many but not necessarily all medical decisions.

Long-term care dermatology is truly its own art form. And it is a growing specialty, drawing from the realm of both dermatology and geriatrics.

Those of us that work in long-term care serve a population composed of over 2.7 million patients. That is the total estimated population in nursing homes and ALFs.

Taler mentions the growing complexity of nursing home care [1].

The prevalence of pressure ulcers (PUs) in long-term care facilities is estimated to be between 2.4 % and 23 % [2] and the incidence of new ulcers over a 6-month period is approximately 12 % [3]. In the 1980s, Smith et al. showed an increasing prevalence of patients being discharged from the hospital with pressure ulcers, attributable to an aging population and the greater complexity and frailty of the patients currently treated in the acute care setting. Due to constraints on hospital utilization, the transfer of patients to nursing homes has resulted in up to 63 % of pressure ulcers present on admission to the facility and increased costs of care [4–7].

Neurodermatitis

Psychiatry-based medications such as doxepin have been routinely prescribed by dermatologists for agitated, itchy patients. For severe neurodermatitis, we are now prescribing medications formerly in the realm of psychiatry, such as olanzapine or risperidone. Dermatologists have been acutely aware for years of the powerful mind-body interactions encountered every day in clinical practice.

Scabies and Norwegian Scabies

Typically, scabies causes intense itching and tracks in the cutaneous layer of the skin, where the mites have burrowed. Certain forms of scabies such as keratotic or crusted variants are problematic in the elderly, especially those who are immunocompromised; their skin may become so thickened that itching may not be present. Scratching serves a purpose in scabies, as some mites are removed by the scratching. When the infested person does not scratch the mites multiply without disruption causing hyperinfestation. People at risk for this type of scabies include those who live in institutions and are physically infirm, have other diseases which affect sensation in the skin such as diabetes, or are taking medications, such as history of treatment with steroids, which lower their immune response.

In typical scabies, the person is infested with approximately 10–15 mites, whereas in crusted scabies, thousands of mites are burrowed in the skin, which increases the potential for transmission.

Nosocomial transmission of scabies occurs primarily through prolonged skin-to-skin contact with someone who is infested. Transmission of scabies with those who have crusted scabies needs only a short period of skin-to skin contact. Staff can acquire scabies while performing resident care such as bathing, lifting, or applying lotions. Mites can only live out of the skin for about 3 days; however, scabies can be passed on during that time through contact with infested clothing or bedding.

Staffs who are exposed to scabies but lack signs of infestation normally do not require prophylactic treatment. In outbreak situations where infestations continue to occur, prophylaxis may be warranted for both residents and exposed staff. Staffs who are infested with scabies should be restricted from hands-on care until after they have received the initial treatment and have been medically evaluated and determined to be free of infestation. Staff should be advised to report for further medical evaluation if symptoms do not subside.

Treatment Recommendations

Keep in mind the seven tips below.

1. Whenever possible, identify the reason for each prescribed medication.

2. Begin treatment with the lowest possible dose and prescribe short courses of treatment. Continually reevaluate the clinical outcome.

3. Assume that the treatment will not be provided as often as prescribed. Workload, time restraints, and poor compliance are all issues which affect the treatment of skin conditions in the long-term care patient. If you prescribe triamcinolone cream 0.1 % for an eczematous dermatitis, I recommend writing it TID with the hope that it will get applied at least once a day.

4. Check on the "prn" or routine medications no longer clinically indicated for a resident and eliminate unnecessary treatments.

5. Work with the nursing staff and attending physician on neuropharmacological agents, checking to make sure that the prescribed drugs do not interfere with current treatments.

6. Do not forget the simple preventions, such as antibacterial soaps, frequent handwashing, proper shoes, supports and devices for wound prevention, adequate hydration and humidity, proper lighting, and eliminating high-fall risks.

7. At least once a year, provide in-services to the nursing home staff on dermatology issues. The staffs acquire CEUs and are generally very appreciative of your time. You are a crucial part of the team in improving the residents' treatment, and face-to-face encounters are crucial in maintaining an ongoing quality of care.

Newer books and articles have addressed the issues of geriatric dermatology and nursing home care. Geriatric dermatology and nursing home care is a very specific specialty and includes xerosis, nutritional deficiencies, elder abuse, and stasis dermatitis. The nursing home specialist must have expertise in the unique structure and function of aging skin and demographic understanding. Wound care measurements and training are important. Integrative techniques must also be considered [8–25].

Dermatologists may be able to increase their involvement in the nursing home population by contacting directors of nursing or administrators and ask about providing services. Dermatology resident physicians would benefit from spending at least a week working in the nursing home setting doing consults. By increasing interactions with the population of older adults in nursing homes, dermatologists are more likely to diagnose and effectively treat skin problems of the elderly, a growing population.

Appendix

Debilitating skin diseases in long-term care facilities cause avoidable pain and suffering. In addition, they place a large additional burden on low budgets. Although most long-term care administrators and staffs recognize the need for improved prevention and management of skin diseases, they lack the necessary time for development of these efforts. A systematic approach using risk assessment tools will prove highly effective to reduce the incidence of debilitating skin diseases in long-term care facilities.

Previous scales and risk assessment tools have been excellent nursing assessment tools for evaluating a patient's general condition, alerting us to the need for increased vigilance. However, inadequate pressure relief and poor recognition by staff are at the very core of pressure ulcer and debilitating skin disease problems. Therefore, I have incorporated an "interactive" component to the risk assessment tool that will include "points" (improved score) for those facilities that maintain adequate surface support and staff training.

Please use this in your facility and provide me with feedback on your efforts. Thank you for helping the elderly and disabled.

DR. NORMAN'S
SKIN CARE ASSESSMENT FORM
(copyright 2001 Dr. Robert A. Norman)

	Dates

MENTAL STATUS & SENSORY PERCEPTION (score)
(Orientation & Ability to respond to pressure

Comments:

1 Oriented and cooperative, no sensory impairment

2 Slightly limited (Responds to verbal commands)

3 Disoriented or confused, unable to communicate and very limited (Responds to painful stimuli)

4 Stuporous, lethargic, or sedated, completely limited sensory perception (Unresponsive)

MOBILITY STATUS (score)
(Ability to change and control body position)

Comments

1 Full (can turn self) with no limitations

2 Slightly limited (Frequent/slight changes)

3 Limited or restrained: has contractures

4 Immobile, insensate

MOISTURE, BOWEL AND BLADDER STATUS (score)

Comments

1 Fully continent, rarely moist

2 Occassionally moist and incontinent of urine, feces (Extra change q day)

3 Very moist (Linen/diaper/pad changed q shift)

4 Constantly moist (moisture detected each time moved--Totally incontinent of urine and feces)

SKIN INTEGRITY & FRICTION TEAR (score)

Comments:

1 Good turgor with no apparent problem (well hydrated, elasticity WNL for age) maintains good position

2 Potential problem--poor turgor (increased fragility, history of skin breakdown, moves feebly/some sliding)

3 Probable problem (history of ulcers, skin tears, severe purpura, severe sun damage, or moderate to severe stasis dermatitis)

4. Problem (Constant friction, existing skin ulcers/lesions)

Resident Name: ____Admission
NO. ______________

NORMAN SCALE

SKIN CARE ASSESSMENT FORM

Dates

ACTIVITY STATUS (SCORE)	

(Ability to change and control body position)

1 Full(can turn self) with no limitations
2 Slightly limited(Frequent/slight changes)
3. Very limited(restrained, has contractures or
  infrequent changes)
4 Completely immobile, insensate(requires assistance
  to move) even if able to watch TV

Comments:

NUTRITIONAL/FLUID STATUS (SCORE)

(Usual food intake & lab parameters)

1 Excellent with IBW, at or above 3.5 serum
  albumin, BUN and Creat WNL, eats well, spoon fed
  or self fed, over 90% acceptance

2 Adequate (>1/2 meal, 4 servings protein, Tube/TPN
  feeding 150% acceptance routinely, above or below
  IBW, albumin, BUN & creat WNL)

3 Probably adequate(<3 servings protein, 1/2 meal &
  BUN/CREAT altered or edema present, above or
  below IBW, albumin at or below 3.5 gm/dl

4 Very Poor (Never completes meal with less than 50%
acceptance routinely/ npo or liquids > 5 days, above
or below IBW with albumin at or below 3.5gm/dl,
BUN/CREAT altered

Comments:

PREDISPOSING MEDICAL PROBLEMS (SCORE)

AND INFLUENCING HEALTH FACTORS:

(score (1) for each present)

(Severe neurodermatitis, Age > 75, recent
Nicotine Abuse of more than 10 pack years,
Low pre-albumin,transferrin, hemoglobin, or zinc;
infection, edema, temperature elevation, dehydration
 COPD, ASCVD, PVD, diabetes, liver or renal disease
cancer, motor or sensory deficits, osteomyelitis,
depression, use of steroids, antipsychotics,
anticoagulants)

(1) One present
(2) Two present
(3) Three present
(4) Four or more present

TOTAL SCORE

10 or under-minimal risk
11-13 low risk
14-15 moderate risk
16 or > high risk

Comments:

comprehensive staff training in wound prevention and care-- subtract (5) five points

support surface (bed) for wound prevention (and wheelchair if needed)--subtract (5) five points

NURSES INITIALS

PAGE 2

Resident Name: ____**Admission NO.**_____________

References

1. Taler G. Management of pressure ulcers in long-term care. Adv Wound Care. 1997;10(5):50–2.
2. Taler G. Pressure ulcers in clinical practice guidelines. Columbia, MD: American Medical Directors Association; 1996.
3. Taler G, Richardson JP, Fredman L, Lazur A. The wound unit: a specialized unit for pressure sore management in a long term care facility. Md Med J. 1994;43:165–9.
4. Smith DM, Winsemius DK, Besdine RW. Pressure sores in the elderly: Can this outcome be improved? J Gen Intern Med. 1991;6:81–93.
5. Olshansky K. Pressure ulcer risk assessment scales—the missing link. Adv Wound Care. 1998;11(2):90.
6. Frantz RA, Gardner S, Harvey P, Specht J. The cost of treating pressure ulcers in a long-term care facility. Decubitus. 1991;4(3):37–45.
7. Xakellis GC, Frantz RA, Lewis AJ. Costs of preventing pressure ulcers in the long term care facility. Am Geriatr Soc. 1995;43:496–501.
8. Norman R. Common skin conditions in geriatric dermatology. Annals Long-Term Care. 2008;16(6):40–5.
9. Norman R, editor. Diagnosis of aging skin diseases. London: Springer Publishing; 2008.
10. Norman R. The demographic imperative in diagnosis of aging skin diseases. London: Springer Publishing; 2008.
11. Norman R, Menendez R. Structure and function of aging skin, in diagnosis of aging skin diseases. London: Springer Publishing; 2008.
12. Norman R. Xerosis and pruritis in the elderly: recognition and management, in diagnosis of aging skin diseases. London: Springer Publishing; 2008.
13. Haight R, Norman R. The cutaneous manifestations of nutritional deficiencies, in diagnosis of aging skin diseases. London: Springer Publishing; 2008.
14. Chakrabarty A, Norman R, Philips T. Cutaneous manifestations of diabetes, in diagnosis of aging skin diseases. London: Springer Publishing; 2008.
15. Norman R. Geriatric dermatology: head to Toe evaluation, in diagnosis of aging skin diseases. London: Springer Publishing; 2008.

16. Norman R, Dewberry C, Bock M. Selected geriatric dermatology case studies, in diagnosis of aging skin diseases. London: Springer Publishing; 2008.
17. Norman R. Effectively manage older patients with skin disease. Pract Dermatol. 2011.
18. Norman R. Clinical cases in geriatric dermatology (With Endo, J.) (December 2012) Springer-Verlag.
19. Endo J, Wong J, Norman R, Chang A. Geriatric dermatology: Part I. Geriatric pharmacology for the dermatologist. J Am Acad Dermatol. 2013;68(521.e1):10.
20. Chang AL, Wong J, Endo J, Norman R. Geriatric dermatology: Part II Risk factors and cutaneous signs of elder mistreatment for the dermatologist. J Am Acad Dermatol. 2013;68(4):533.e1–10.
21. Chang AL, Wong JW, Endo JO, Norman RA. Geriatric dermatology review: major changes in skin function in older patients and their contribution to common clinical challenges. J Am Med Dir Assoc. 2013;14(10):724–30.
22. Norman R, Young E. Atlas of geriatric dermatology. London: Springer-Verlag; 2013.
23. Dr. Norman's Skin Care Assessment Form 2001.
24. Norman R. Integrative management of skin cancer. In: Norman R et al., editors. Integrative dermatology. New York: Oxford University Press; 2014. p. 425–33. 25.
25. Norman R, Brennan P. Integrative management of stasis dermatitis. In: Norman R et al., editors. Integrative dermatology. New York: Oxford University Press; 2014. p. 434–8. 26.

Evidence-Based Treatment of Actinic Keratoses in Older Adults

Shannon Famenini, Nason Azizi, Andy Liu, and Anne Lynn S. Chang

Introduction

Actinic keratoses (AKs) are cutaneous lesions characterized by proliferation of atypical epidermal keratinocytes in response to chronic exposure to sunlight. They present as erythematous, scaly papules on sun-exposed areas that commonly include the balding scalp, face, neck, dorsal hands, and forearms. AKs can progress to squamous cell carcinoma (SCC). The likelihood of conversion has been estimated to occur at a rate of 0.075–0.096 % per lesion per year [1]. Other estimates are even higher with rates of 13–20 % over a 10-year period if lesions are left untreated. The progression of AK to SCC is estimated to take from 10 to 20 years [2], with more rapid progression in immunosuppressed individuals. Because AKs represent the initial stage in the evolution of squamous cell carcinoma, they are typically treated, although spontaneous regression has been observed to occur at a rate of 15–63 % per year, with recurrence rates of 15–53 % [3]. AKs are typically diagnosed on clinical exam by visual inspection and a gritty texture on palpation.

Epidemiology

The prevalence of AK increases with age. Among Caucasians it has been reported that prevalence rates are less than 10 % for individuals in their third decade of life but more than 80 % in their seventh decade [4]. Men are at increased risk for developing AKs, most likely due to occupational and recreational exposure. In the UK, prevalence of AK for individuals between the ages 16 and 49 years was found to be 27 % for males and 13 % for females, a little more than double the prevalence for males. However, in the age group from 50 to 86 years, prevalence was more evenly distributed between sexes, 66 % for males and 56 % for females. In Brazil, a cohort of Japanese-Brazilians were diagnosed with AK at a mean age of 68.9 years [5].

AKs represent one of the top three most frequent reasons for consulting a dermatologist [4]. Between 1990 and 1999, AKs were diagnosed in

S. Famenini, M.D.
David Getier School of Medicine, 10503 Woodfield Court, Los Angeles, CA 90077, USA

N. Azizi, M.D.
Department of Dermatology, Stanford University School of Medicine, 450 Broadway Street, MC5334, Redwood City, CA 94063, USA
e-mail: alschang@stanford.edu

A.L.S. Chang, M.D. (✉)
Assistant Professor, Department of Dermatology, Stanford University School of Medicine, 450 Broadway Street, MC5334, Redwood City, CA 94063, USA
e-mail: alschang@stanford.edu

A. Liu, B.S.
Albert Einstein College of Medicine, 1300 Morris Park Ave., Bronx, NY 10461, USA

© Springer International Publishing Switzerland 2015
A.L.S. Chang (ed.), *Advances in Geriatric Dermatology*, DOI 10.1007/978-3-319-18380-0_8

47 million visits, or 14 % of all visits to the dermatologist's office [6]. They are primarily seen in fair-skinned individuals who have had long-term sun exposure. Sun-sensitive cutaneous phenotypes include people who are fair skinned, have light-colored eyes, and have red or blond hair. In addition, the inability to tan, tendency to sunburn easily, and ability to form freckles are consistent with this phenotype [4]. In one study, prevalence rates were reported to be as high as 40–50 % in Australian residents older than 40 years; individuals with fair skin had a relative risk of 14.1 when compared with persons of olive skin color, and individuals with medium skin color had a 6.5-fold relative risk [7]. In the USA, lower prevalence rates have been reported ranging from 11 to 26 % [4]. In darker skinned individuals, AKs are extremely rare. Cumulative ultraviolet radiation is the other major risk factor for AKs. The frequency of AKs is greater in residents of sunny countries closer to the equator and those with outdoor occupations [7, 8]. In fact, one study showed that individuals with maximal occupational UV light exposure had an increase in relative risk of 2.4; those with multiple AKs were 4.3 times as likely to have maximal occupational UV light exposure [4].

Molecular Understanding

Normally, melanin in the epidermis absorbs UV and protects keratinocytes from DNA damage. Overexposure to UV radiation induces a mutation in the p53 tumor-suppressor gene (single-nucleotide substitutions at a dipyrimidine site: C to T, C to A, or T to C). This mutation inhibits the cell's ability to undergo apoptosis, which leads to atypical proliferation of keratinocytes in the epidermis, and ultimately AK [9].

Prevention

Protection from UV radiation reduces the risk for developing AK. Patients are commonly recommended to avoid sunlight or seek shade during midday hours when UV exposure is greatest.

Patients are also encouraged to use protective clothing, such as hats, long-sleeved clothing, and sunglasses. Importantly, the regular use of sunscreen prevents the development of AKs. In a randomized, controlled trial published in the New England Journal of Medicine it was shown that people 40 years and older who used SPF 17 sunscreen for only 1 month had fewer new AK lesions and more remissions. In fact, the mean number of AKs decreased by 0.6 in the sunscreen group [10].

Treatment

Because AKs represent the initial stage in the evolution of squamous cell carcinoma, recognition and treatment are important. Treatment is administered based on characteristics and number of lesions, patient preference for the mode and duration of treatment, willingness and ability to comply with self-administered therapies, as well as tolerance of side effects. In older patients with poor vision, memory, or manual dexterity, a caregiver may need to be enlisted to apply topical pharmacotherapy.

One consideration in selecting the treatment modality for AKs is treatment efficacy. Comparison of treatment efficacy across studies should account for follow-up times after treatment across, outcomes assessed, a number of treatment cycles, and severity of disease treated.

The most widely utilized treatment for AKs in the office is liquid nitrogen cryotherapy because it is quick, is easily performed in the office setting, produces excellent cosmetic results, and is well tolerated by patients. It is considered the standard of care and particularly useful when lesions are scattered or few in number [11]. This technique uses liquid nitrogen to freeze and destroy the epidermis containing AK with an efficacy cure rate as high as 98.9 % after 1 year [12]. In a review written for the Cochrane Collaboration, the use of cryotherapy was evaluated against other treatment options for AK. They report that a 1-week course of topical 0.5 % 5-fluorouracil (5-FU) before cryosurgery resulted in significantly less AKs 6 months after treatment than cryosurgery alone. Similarly, combination therapy with imiquimod is more efficacious when compared to cryotherapy alone [13]. One of the drawbacks of using cryotherapy however is the inability to preserve tissue for histologic analysis to rule out other neoplasms such as squamous cell carcinoma. In addition, thick lesions and lesions on the dorsum of hand do not respond as well [14]. The main side effects of cryotherapy include burning and stinging during treatment and possible hypopigmentation following treatment [15]. Pain associated with cryotherapy is usually well tolerated but not insignificant. One study surveying patient response to pain found levels to be higher than deemed appropriate by patients but below levels necessary for additional analgesics; only 30.4 % reported the need for prior analgesia and 69.9 % reported no need for analgesia [16]. In older patients with areas of thinner skin, cryotherapy may be effective with reduced thaw times, although this has not been formally studied.

In patients with multiple lesions localized in the same area such as on the face or arms, topical pharmacotherapy is an effective alternative to spot treatment with cryotherapy, in part due to their visibility to the patient for applying the medication. A critical concern in older adults who are prescribed topical field therapy is to make sure that patients have adequate visual acuity to identify the target lesion and the manual dexterity to apply the medication to the required site(s). The FDA-approved topical treatments include 5-FU, imiquimod, diclofenac, and ingenol mebutate as well as several off-label options.

Of these, 5-FU is the most widely used. 5-FU works by inhibiting thymidylate synthetase, the enzyme normally responsible for conversion of deoxyuridine 5-monophosphate (DUMP) to thymidine 5-monophosphate (TMP), which ultimately inhibits DNA synthesis [17]. This mode of treatment preferentially targets AKs with minimal effects on normal skin [18]. Inflammation of AK lesions typically occurs within 2 weeks of initiating therapy and serves as visual evidence that lesion destruction is occurring which may cause irritation and discomfort in some patients [19]. It is important to educate patients that inflamma-

tion, erythema, blistering, and re-epithelialization are to be expected in order to promote therapy compliance and prevent premature discontinuation of therapy. Lesion response rates were reported to be 87.8 % in one meta-analysis of seven studies [20]. There is ongoing analysis demonstrating that lower dose, once-daily 0.5 % 5-FU may be more tolerable, safer, cost effective, and equally as efficacious as 5 % 5-FU [21, 22]. In a patient population where treatment compliance is low [23], the reduction of irritability and improvement in adverse events may increase adherence to the regimen [19]. In a review of nine studies following standard treatment regimens comparing complete clearance rates, results for 0.5 % and 5 % 5-FU ranged from 16.7 to 57.8 % and 43 to 100 %, respectively [24]. There is a need for additional comparative studies since tolerability rates among studies were unable to be compared. In one study where each patient received both treatments (5 % twice daily and 0.5 % once daily) on each side of their face, both treatments achieved 43 % complete clearance rates [25]. Patients in that trial preferred the lower dose fluorouracil.

Imiquimod is another popular topical pharmacotherapy that works by modulating the immune response. It binds to cell surface receptors such as Toll-like receptor 7 [26] and induces the synthesis of interferon-alpha and other cytokines that have antitumor properties [27]. Therapeutic skin responses include erythema and crusting but therapy is well tolerated [28, 29]. In a study comparing 5-FU and imiquimod, tolerability was similar between the two treatments. Erythema was more prominent in patients receiving 5-FU initially, but by week 16, erythematous lesions became less prominent than those seen with imiquimod therapy [30]. Complete clearance is expected in 50 % of patients [31]. Recent studies investigating the lower doses of imiquimod, 2.5 and 3.75 % versus the traditional 5 % cream, suggest comparable efficacy [32, 33] and potential benefits in tolerability [34].

Ingenol mebutate is the newest addition to the arsenal for the treatment of AK. Derived from the sap of the plant *Euphorbia peplus*, ingenol mebutate was approved by the FDA in

2012. It is touted to operate via two mechanisms of action: rapid lesion necrosis and specific neutrophil-mediated, antibody-dependent cellular cytotoxicity [35]. Owing to the rapid cytotoxic response and degradation of plasma membrane, the treatment period is 2–3 days. Studies find complete clearance rates in 42.2 % in lesions involving the face and scalp and 34.1 % in lesions involving the trunk and extremities [36]. Side effects including erythema, flaking, and crusting are described to be mild to moderate and resolve in 2 and 4 weeks for the face/scalp and trunk/extremities, respectively [37]. A long-term, 12-month follow-up study found reduction in the number of AKs by 87 % [38].

A valuable modality for field treatment in older adults is photodynamic therapy (PDT), because it does not require the patient to self-apply medication to the correct lesions. This is therefore a good choice for older adults with visual, cognitive, or manual dexterity issues. PDT employs the use of topical photosensitization followed by visible light irradiation to the affected area of skin. The ensuing photochemical activation destroys cells [39]. Two commonly used sensitizing agents include 5-aminolevulinic acid (ALA) and methyl aminolevulinate (MAL), the former used widely in the USA. Overall, PDT is highly effective in treating AKs. Three-month complete response rates for MAL-PDT and ALA-PDT are 90 % and 91 %, respectively [40, 41]. One of the disadvantages to PDT is the pain during illumination. In a retrospective study of 24 patients, all patients reported moderate or severe pain (42 % and 58 %, respectively) during photo irradiation [42]. In a study that aimed at identifying important factors of pain during PDT, researchers found that the greater the erythema, the greater the pain reported, but also the better the outcome [43]. In comparison with 5-FU and cryotherapy, ALA/MAL-PDT treatment appears more effective and may result in a better cosmetic outcome [13]. PDT treatment followed by imiquimod achieves significantly better results than either one alone; better tolerance and less intense local reactions are also reported [44]. One study shows that the use of long-pulsed dye laser

(LP PDL) following ALA application minimizes pain during light treatment and achieves comparable efficacy [45, 46].

Recently, a systematic review and meta-analysis of four PDT versus cryotherapy studies (all with mean ages of participants exceeding 64 years) demonstrated a 14 % increased likelihood of complete lesion clearance than cryotherapy at 3 months after treatment [47]. Nevertheless, PDT is limited by availability of equipment, trained staff to apply the dye, and willingness of patient to devote time for incubation and subsequent posttreatment avoidance of sun exposure.

Because the data on treatments for AKs is limited by lack of direct comparison between some interventions, a novel network meta-analysis was performed for common treatments that were randomized controlled trials in non-immunosuppressed participants with mean ages all exceeding 59 years [48]. The results showed that efficacy was highest for 5-FU 0.5 or 5 % > ALA-PDT > cryotherapy > diclofenac 3 %/hyaluronic acid > imiquimod 5 % > ingenol 0.15–0.05 %. This study showed that efficacy was independent of anatomic location except for ingenol.

Second-line topical therapies for actinic keratosis include diclofenac and retinoids and can be considered in older patients who declined first-line treatments topical pharmacotherapies outlined above. They can be used between regular visits for cryotherapy.

Diclofenac is a nonsteroidal anti-inflammatory topical cream approved for use on AKs. While the exact mechanism of action is unknown, it is hypothesized that anti-inflammatory COX-2 inhibition, inhibition of angiogenesis, and induction of apoptosis are responsible for its effect [49, 50]. Compared with the aforementioned topical creams, the treatment period for diclofenac is slightly longer, 60–90 days, a potential disadvantage for this mode of therapy. Complete clearance is recorded in only 40 % of patients [51]. Diclofenac is reported to induce milder inflammation compared with 5-FU [52]. A Cochrane collaboration analysis of interventions for AKs published in 2012 reported that among topical pharmacotherapies, the highest number of participants withdrawing from treatment due to adverse events with highest with 3 % diclofenac compared to imiquimod 5 % [13].

Retinoids are synthetic or natural analogues of vitamin A known to have antineoplastic effects [53]. An analysis of double-blind studies at 31 sites for a total of 1,265 patients found significant reductions in lesions treated with tretinoin (56 %) compared to control (41 %) [54]. In contrast, data from the Veterans Affairs Topical Tretinoin Chemoprevention Trial randomizing 1,131 patients to 0.1 % tretinoin or a vehicle found no statistical significant in AK counts [55]. Adapalene, a third-generation synthetic retinoid, exhibits selectivity for the nuclear retinoic acid receptor, resulting in increased anti-inflammatory activity while inducing less irritation [56]. In a randomized trial, patients treated with 0.1 % and 0.3 % adapalene gel experienced a reduction in the mean number of AKs by 0.5 and 2.5, respectively [57].

Other therapies in dermatology have also been studied in the treatment of AKs. These include using CO_2 and Er:YAG ablative resurfacing lasers. A prospective study of 55 patients (mean age 72.8 years) treated with either topical 5-FU or erbium:yttrium-aluminum-garnet (Er:YAG) laser resurfacing found significantly lower rates of recurrence after 1 year [58]. However, increased erythema, edema, and infections were seen in the laser therapy group. Ablative resurfacing with carbon dioxide lasers in the treatment of AKs was compared with fluorouracil and trichloroacetic acid (TCA); all three groups performed significantly better than the control group, resulting in an 83–92 % reduction in AKs [59]. No significant differences were found among the groups and further studies are needed to assess the efficacy of resurfacing lasers. While laser therapy is more expensive than topical pharmacotherapy, it is possible that overall costs may be lower if fewer recurrences occur in individuals with widespread AKs.

For large areas affected by multiple lesions such as on the scalp or forehead, dermabrasion has been utilized when topical treatments are not appropriate. The technique involves sanding away the stratum corneum under anesthesia, which leaves the residual skin red and painful. A small retrospective study of 23 patients revealed that 96 % remained free from new AKs after 1 year and 83 % clear at 2 years, and an average recurrence time of 4 years [60]. The authors concluded that dermabrasion is an effective longer term prophylaxis compared with other treatments; however more studies are required to confirm this.

A chemical peel is a procedure in which a topical solution is used to injure the skin to a particular depth. This stimulates cell regrowth and even melanin distribution [61]. The Monheit's combination consists of Jessner's solution (resorcinol, lactic acid, and salicylic acid) with TCA and is used for a medium-depth peel [62]. While a superficial peel agent like glycolic acid targets the epidermal/dermal border, the medium-depth peel disturbs the deeper papillary dermis. Care should be taken to prevent scarring in this layer. Side effects include stinging, peeling lasting approximately 1 week, and potential pigmentation changes. In 15 patients where 35 % TCA and Jessner's solution was compared with topical 5-FU, the number of AKs in both groups was reduced by 75 % [63]. Though the results were similar, patients preferred the peel to 5-FU because of its singular application and decreased morbidity. A separate study found no significant differences between the two treatments in long-term efficacy and recommended yearly reevaluations [64].

Treatment Preferences

In a random national sample of 293 dermatologists and 241 primary care providers, researchers looked at 1,743 AK patients (of which 59 % were aged 65 years or older) and reported cryotherapy as the sole form of treatment in 74.6 % of patients, while pharmacotherapy was utilized in only 16.3 % of patients [65]. In multivariate analysis, patients above the age of 65 years were 37 % less likely to receive pharmacotherapy ($p < 0.05$), although the reasons are unclear. Although patient preference was not examined specifically in the age 65 or older group, overall, a majority of patients preferred topical pharmacotherapy rather than cryotherapy, likely due to the discomfort and potential anxiety associated with routine visits. Physicians in general preferred cryotherapy over pharmacotherapy, and dissonance between patient and physician preferences was greater when the dermatologist was the provider versus a primary care provider. In another study of patient perceptions of treatment satisfaction and outcomes in which 39 patients (80 % of whom were older than 60 years) were asked to report their preferences, PDT was significantly preferred to 5-FU or imiquimod [66]. Further studies are needed to catalog elderly patient preferences. Given the range of available treatments for AKs, a discussion of the pros and cons of each treatment modality should occur to identify the best one for the older adult.

References

1. Marks R, Rennie G, Selwood TS. Malignant transformation of solar keratoses to squamous cell carcinoma. Lancet. 1988;1:795–7.
2. Rigel DS, Cockerell CJ, Carucci J, Wharton J. Actinic keratosis, basal cell carcinoma and squamous cell carcinoma. In: Bolognia JL, Jorizzo JL, Rapini RP, editors. Bolognia textbook of dermatology. 2nd ed. Spain: Mosby Elsevier; 2008. p. 1645.
3. Werner R, Sammain A, Erdmann R, Hartmann V, Stockfleth E, Nast A. The natural history of actinic keratosis: a systematic review. Br J Dermatol. 2013;169:502–18.
4. Salasche SJ. Epidemiology of actinic keratoses and squamous cell carcinoma. J Am Acad Dermatol. 2000;42:4–7.
5. Ishioka P, Marques SA, Hirai AT, Marques ME, Hirata SH, Yamada S. Prevalence of precancerous skin lesions and non-melanoma skin cancer in Japanese-Brazilians in Bauru, Sao Paulo State, Brazil. Cad Saude Publica. 2009;25:965–71.
6. Feldman SR, Fleischer Jr AB, McConnell RC. Most common dermatologic problems identified by internists, 1990–1994. Arch Intern Med. 1998;158:726–30.
7. Frost CA, Green AC, Williams GM. The prevalence and determinants of solar keratoses at a subtropical latitude (Queensland, Australia). Br J Dermatol. 1998;139:1033–9.
8. Vitasa BC, Taylor HR, Strickland PT, Rosenthal FS, West S, Abbey H, et al. Association of nonmelanoma skin cancer and actinic keratosis with cumulative solar ultraviolet exposure in Maryland watermen. Cancer. 1990;65:2811–7.
9. Ziegler A, Jonason AS, Leffell DJ, Simon JA, Sharma HW, Kimmelman J, et al. Sunburn and p53 in the onset of skin cancer. Nature. 1994;372:773–6.
10. Thompson SC, Jolley D, Marks R. Reduction of solar keratoses by regular sunscreen use. N Engl J Med. 1993;329:1147–51.
11. Goldberg LH, Kaplan B, Vergilis-Kalner I, Landau J. Liquid nitrogen: temperature control in the treatment of actinic keratosis. Dermatol Surg. 2010;36:1956–61.
12. Lubritz RR, Smolewski SA. Cryosurgery cure rate of actinic keratoses. J Am Acad Dermatol. 1982;7:631–2.
13. Gupta AK, Paquet M, Villanueva E, Brintnell W. Interventions for actinic keratoses. Cochrane Database Syst Rev. 2012;12, Cd004415.
14. Jeffes III EW, Tang EH. Actinic keratosis. Current treatment options. Am J Clin Dermatol. 2000;1:167–79.
15. Thai KE, Fergin P, Freeman M, Vinciullo C, Francis D, Spelman L, et al. A prospective study of the use of cryosurgery for the treatment of actinic keratoses. Int J Dermatol. 2004;43:687–92.
16. Poziomczyk CS, Koche B, Dornelles Mde A, Dornelles SI. Pain evaluation in the cryosurgery of actinic keratoses. An Bras Dermatol. 2011;86:645–50.
17. Eaglstein WH, Weinstein GD, Frost P. Fluorouracil: mechanism of action in human skin and actinic keratoses. I. Effect on DNA synthesis in vivo. Arch Dermatol. 1970;101:132–9.
18. Weinberg JM. Topical therapy for actinic keratoses: current and evolving therapies. Rev Recent Clin Trials. 2006;1:53–60.
19. Werschler WP. Considerations for use of Fluorouracil cream 0.5 % for the treatment of actinic keratosis in elderly patients. J Clin Aesthet Dermatol. 2008;1:22–7.
20. Gupta AK. The management of actinic keratoses in the United States with topical fluorouracil: a pharmacoeconomic evaluation. Cutis. 2002;70:30–6.
21. Stough D, Bucko AD, Vamvakias G, Rafal ES, Davis SA. Fluorouracil cream 0.5 % for actinic keratoses on multiple body sites: an 18-month open-label study. Cutis. 2010;85:267–73.
22. Jorizzo JL, Carney PS, Ko WT, Robins P, Weinkle SH, Werschler WP. Fluorouracil 5 % and 0.5 % creams for the treatment of actinic keratosis: equivalent efficacy with a lower concentration and more convenient dosing schedule. Cutis. 2004;74:18–23.
23. Salzman C. Medication compliance in the elderly. J Clin Psychiatry. 1995;56 Suppl 1:18–22. discussion 3.
24. Kaur RR, Alikhan A, Maibach HI. Comparison of topical 5-fluorouracil formulations in actinic keratosis treatment. J Dermatolog Treat. 2010;21:267–71.
25. Loven K, Stein L, Furst K, Levy S. Evaluation of the efficacy and tolerability of 0.5 % fluorouracil cream and 5 % fluorouracil cream applied to each side of the

face in patients with actinic keratosis. Clin Ther. 2002;24:990–1000.

26. Hemmi H, Kaisho T, Takeuchi O, Sato S, Sanjo H, Hoshino K, et al. Small anti-viral compounds activate immune cells via the TLR7 MyD88-dependent signaling pathway. Nat Immunol. 2002;3:196–200.

27. Stanley MA. Imiquimod and the imidazoquinolones: mechanism of action and therapeutic potential. Clin Exp Dermatol. 2002;27:571–7.

28. Stockfleth E, Meyer T, Benninghoff B, Salasche S, Papadopoulos L, Ulrich C, et al. A randomized, double-blind, vehicle-controlled study to assess 5 % imiquimod cream for the treatment of multiple actinic keratoses. Arch Dermatol. 2002;138:1498–502.

29. Strohal R, Kerl H, Schuster L. Treatment of actinic keratoses with 5 % topical imiquimod: a multicenter prospective observational study from 93 Austrian office-based dermatologists. J Drugs Dermatol. 2012; 11:574–8.

30. Tanghetti E, Werschler P. Comparison of 5 % 5-fluorouracil cream and 5 % imiquimod cream in the management of actinic keratoses on the face and scalp. J Drugs Dermatol. 2007;6:144–7.

31. Hadley G, Derry S, Moore RA. Imiquimod for actinic keratosis: systematic review and meta-analysis. J Invest Dermatol. 2006;126:1251–5.

32. Swanson N, Abramovits W, Berman B, Kulp J, Rigel DS, Levy S. Imiquimod 2.5 % and 3.75 % for the treatment of actinic keratoses: results of two placebo-controlled studies of daily application to the face and balding scalp for two 2-week cycles. J Am Acad Dermatol. 2010;62:582–90.

33. Hanke CW, Swanson N, Bruce S, Berman B, Kulp J, Levy S. Complete clearance is sustained for at least 12 months after treatment of actinic keratoses of the face or balding scalp via daily dosing with imiquimod 3.75 % or 2.5 % cream. J Drugs Dermatol. 2011;10: 165–70.

34. Hanke CW, Beer KR, Stockfleth E, Wu J, Rosen T, Levy S. Imiquimod 2.5 % and 3.75 % for the treatment of actinic keratoses: results of two placebo-controlled studies of daily application to the face and balding scalp for two 3-week cycles. J Am Acad Dermatol. 2010;62:573–81.

35. Rosen RH, Gupta AK, Tyring SK. Dual mechanism of action of ingenol mebutate gel for topical treatment of actinic keratoses: rapid lesion necrosis followed by lesion-specific immune response. J Am Acad Dermatol. 2012;66:486–93.

36. Lebwohl M, Swanson N, Anderson LL, Melgaard A, Xu Z, Berman B. Ingenol mebutate gel for actinic keratosis. N Engl J Med. 2012;366:1010–9.

37. Martin G, Swanson N. Clinical findings using ingenol mebutate gel to treat actinic keratoses. J Am Acad Dermatol. 2013;68:S39–48.

38. Lebwohl M, Shumack S, Gold L, Melgaard A, Larsson T, Tyring SK. Long-term follow-up study of ingenol mebutate gel for the treatment of actinic keratoses. JAMA Dermatol. 2013;149:666–70.

39. Ericson MB, Wennberg AM, Larko O. Review of photodynamic therapy in actinic keratosis and basal cell carcinoma. Ther Clin Risk Manag. 2008;4:1–9.

40. Braathen LR, Szeimies RM, Basset-Seguin N, Bissonnette R, Foley P, Pariser D, et al. Guidelines on the use of photodynamic therapy for nonmelanoma skin cancer: an international consensus. International Society for Photodynamic Therapy in Dermatology, 2005. J Am Acad Dermatol. 2007;56:125–43.

41. Jeffes EW, McCullough JL, Weinstein GD, Fergin PE, Nelson JS, Shull TF, et al. Photodynamic therapy of actinic keratosis with topical 5-aminolevulinic acid. A pilot dose-ranging study. Arch Dermatol. 1997;133: 727–32.

42. Tran DT, Salmon R. Field treatment of facial and scalp actinic keratoses with photodynamic therapy: survey of patient perceptions of treatment satisfaction and outcomes. Australas J Dermatol. 2011;52: 195–201.

43. Sandberg C, Stenquist B, Rosdahl I, Ros AM, Synnerstad I, Karlsson M, et al. Important factors for pain during photodynamic therapy for actinic keratosis. Acta Derm Venereol. 2006;86:404–8.

44. Serra-Guillen C, Nagore E, Hueso L, Traves V, Messeguer F, Sanmartín O, et al. A randomized pilot comparative study of topical methyl aminolevulinate photodynamic therapy versus imiquimod 5 % versus sequential application of both therapies in immunocompetent patients with actinic keratosis: clinical and histologic outcomes. J Am Acad Dermatol. 2012;66: e131–7.

45. Alexiades-Armenakas MR, Geronemus RG. Laser-mediated photodynamic therapy of actinic keratoses. Arch Dermatol. 2003;139:1313–20.

46. Alexiades-Armenakas M. Laser-mediated photodynamic therapy. Clin Dermatol. 2006;24:16–25.

47. Patel G, Armstrong A, DB E. Efficacy of photodynamic therapy vs other interventions in randomized clinical trials for the treatment of actinic keratosis: a systematic review and meta-analysis. JAMA Dermatol. 2014;150:1281–8.

48. Gupta A, Paquet M. Network meta-analysis of the outcome 'participant complete clearance' in nonimmunosuppressed participants of eight interventions for actinic keratosis: a follow-up on a Cochrane review. Br J Dermatol. 2013;169:250–9.

49. Martin GM, Stockfleth E. Diclofenac sodium 3 % gel for the management of actinic keratosis: 10+ years of cumulative evidence of efficacy and safety. J Drugs Dermatol. 2012;11:600–8.

50. Maltusch A, Röwert-Huber J, Matthies C, Lange-Asschenfeldt S, Stockfleth E. Modes of action of diclofenac 3 %/hyaluronic acid 2.5 % in the treatment of actinic keratosis. J Dtsch Dermatol Ges. 2011;9: 1011–7.

51. Pirard D, Vereecken P, Melot C, Heenen M. Three percent diclofenac in 2.5 % hyaluronan gel in the treatment of actinic keratoses: a meta-analysis of the recent studies. Arch Dermatol Res. 2005;297:185–9.

52. Smith SR, Morhenn VB, Piacquadio DJ. Bilateral comparison of the efficacy and tolerability of 3 % diclofenac sodium gel and 5 % 5-fluorouracil cream in the treatment of actinic keratoses of the face and scalp. J Drugs Dermatol. 2006;5:156–9.

53. Heller EH, Shiffman NJ. Synthetic retinoids in dermatology. Can Med Assoc J. 1985;132:1129–36.

54. Thorne EG. Long-term clinical experience with a topical retinoid. Br J Dermatol. 1992;127:31–6.

55. Weinstock MA, Bingham SF, Digiovanna JJ, Rizzo AE, Marcolivio K, Hall R, et al. Tretinoin and the prevention of keratinocyte carcinoma (Basal and squamous cell carcinoma of the skin): a veterans affairs randomized chemoprevention trial. J Invest Dermatol. 2012;132:1583–90.

56. Mukherjee S, Date A, Patravale V, Korting HC, Roeder A, Weindl G. Retinoids in the treatment of skin aging: an overview of clinical efficacy and safety. Clin Interv Aging. 2006;1:327–48.

57. Kang S, Goldfarb MT, Weiss JS, Metz RD, Hamilton TA, Voorhees JJ, et al. Assessment of adapalene gel for the treatment of actinic keratoses and lentigines: a randomized trial. J Am Acad Dermatol. 2003;49:83–90.

58. Ostertag JU, Quaedvlieg PJ, van der Geer S, Nelemans P, Christianen ME, Neumann MH, et al. A clinical comparison and long-term follow-up of topical 5-fluorouracil versus laser resurfacing in the treatment of widespread actinic keratoses. Lasers Surg Med. 2006;38:731–9.

59. Hantash BM, Stewart DB, Cooper ZA, Rehmus WE, Koch R, Swetter SM. Facial resurfacing for nonmelanoma skin cancer prophylaxis. Arch Dermatol. 2006;142:976–82.

60. Coleman III WP, Yarborough JM, Mandy SH. Dermabrasion for prophylaxis and treatment of actinic keratoses. Dermatol Surg. 1996;22:17–21.

61. Rendon MI, Berson DS, Cohen JL, Roberts WE, Starker I, Wang B. Evidence and considerations in the application of chemical peels in skin disorders and aesthetic resurfacing. J Clin Aesthet Dermatol. 2010;3:32–43.

62. Monheit GD. The Jessner's-trichloroacetic acid peel. An enhanced medium-depth chemical peel. Dermatol Clin. 1995;13:277–83.

63. Lawrence N, Cox SE, Cockerell CJ, Freeman RG, Cruz Jr PD. A comparison of the efficacy and safety of Jessner's solution and 35 % trichloroacetic acid vs 5 % fluorouracil in the treatment of widespread facial actinic keratoses. Arch Dermatol. 1995;131:176–81.

64. Witheiler DD, Lawrence N, Cox SE, Cruz C, Cockerell CJ, Freemen RG. Long-term efficacy and safety of Jessner's solution and 35 % trichloroacetic acid vs 5 % fluorouracil in the treatment of widespread facial actinic keratoses. Dermatol Surg. 1997;23:191–6.

65. Balkrishnan R, Cayce KA, Kulkarni AS, Orsagh T, Gallagher JR, Richmond D, et al. Predictors of treatment choices and associated outcomes in actinic keratoses: results from a national physician survey study. J Dermatolog Treat. 2006;17:162–6.

66. Tierney EP, Eide MJ, Jacobsen G, Ozog D. Photodynamic therapy for actinic keratoses: survey of patient perceptions of treatment satisfaction and outcomes. J Cosmet Laser Ther. 2008;10:81–6.

Recent Advances in Skin Cancer Treatment in Older Adults

Anne Lynn S. Chang

Introduction

This chapter focuses on new developments in treatment for the three most common cancers in older adults, basal cell carcinoma (BCC), squamous cell carcinoma (SCC), and melanoma. The rate of skin cancers is well known to increase with age. For instance, melanoma demonstrates a dramatic rise after the age of 50 years, especially in men (Fig. 1). In fact, the rate of melanoma in US men appears to double from age 60s to age 80s. According to the National Cancer Institute's Surveillance, Epidemiology and End Results 1975–2011 database, death rates from melanoma increase with age, from 6 % below age 65 years to over 18 % above age 80 years. The rate of non-melanoma skin cancer also rises with age, and recent data shows that larger size of BCC also associates with age [1]. Other new data shows that non-melanoma skin cancer in transplant patients also associates with increasing age [2].

Notable progress has recently been made in new therapies available to individuals with unresectable skin cancer. For instance, targeted therapies such as inhibitors of the Hedgehog pathway

A.L.S. Chang, M.D. (✉)
Assistant Professor, Department of Dermatology,
Stanford University School of Medicine,
450 Broadway Street, MC5334,
Redwood City, CA 94063, USA
e-mail: alschang@stanford.edu

for advanced BCC [3] or BRAF inhibitors for melanomas [4] have resulted in increased survival times in these patients, the median ages of which were over 50 years old in these studies. A different strategy using immunotherapy to unleash the immune response against unresectable or metastatic melanoma utilizes checkpoint inhibitors such as PD1 or PDL1 inhibitors and holds promise for extending survival [5]. Use of these inhibitors in non-melanoma skin cancers remains to be tested in clinical trials.

Basal Cell Carcinoma in Older Adults

A wide range of treatments are available to treat stage I and II BCCs, ranging from excision, Mohs micrographic surgery, radiation, electrodesiccation and curettage, photodynamic therapy, and topical 5-fluorouracil, or imiquimod. These therapies have differing cure rates, modes of delivery, and side effects that factor into selecting the best treatment for the older adult. Randomized studies with cure rates compared to excision, adapted from the National Cancer Institute 2014, are presented in Table 1. Recent data from Australia showed that excision rate was highest for keratinocytic cancers in men aged 75–84 years, and that excision rates declined for individuals less than 45 years [10].

Topical pharmacotherapy for skin cancer is a consideration for individuals who decline or

A.L.S. Chang (ed.), *Advances in Geriatric Dermatology*, DOI 10.1007/978-3-319-18380-0_9

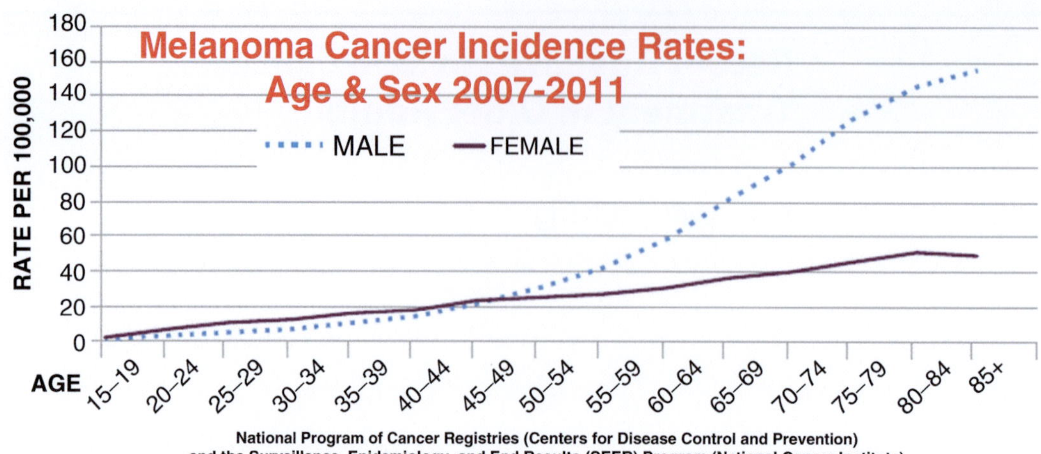

Fig. 1 Melanoma cancer incidence rates 2007–2011 (http://seer.cancer.gov/statfacts/html/melan.html)

Table 1 Cure rates from randomized trials of non-advanced BCC treatments comparing excision to other treatments

Treatments compared	Mean age, years	Recurrence rate	Follow-up time point	Cosmesis	Reference
Excision versus radiation	66	0.7 vs. 7.5 %	4 years	Better with excision	Petit et al. [6]
Excision versus Mohs micrographic surgery	68	3 vs. 2 %	30 months	Similar	Smeets et al. [7]
Excision versus photodynamic therapy (red light ×2 treatments)	68	4 vs. 17 %	12 months	Better with excision	Rhodes et al. [8]
Excision versus cryotherapy	NA	0 vs. 6 %	12 months	Better after excision	Thissen et al. [9]

cannot undergo surgical procedures. Topical 5-fluorouracil (5-FU) 5 % and imiquimod 5 % are FDA approved for small superficial BCCs. While level 1 evidence (according to the Oxford 2011 Levels of Evidence) exists for topical imiquimod use in superficial BCC, only level 2 evidence for topical 5-FU exists for superficial BCC. The largest study to date for 5FU and superficial BCC is a 31-patient study in which 90 % clearance rate was achieved after 11 weeks of twice-daily treatment, with average follow-up time of only 3 weeks [11]. Evidence for 5FU against nodular BCC is level 4 only [12]. Imiquimod has demonstrated utility against superficial and nodular BCC (level 1 and 2 evidence, respectively), with histologic cure rates exceeding 70 % and optimal treatment results

balancing efficacy with tolerability at five applications per week [12]. Nevertheless, follow-up times are limited to 12 weeks or less, and further study is needed to document long-term cure rates [13–17]. More recently, ingenol mebutate has demonstrated level 2 evidence against superficial BCCs [12]. Because of the limited number of studies and short follow-up times in the studies, these topical therapies are generally considered only when patients decline or cannot undergo surgical treatments.

Self-applied topical therapies such as 5-fluorouracil or imiquimod may be difficult for older adults if they are not in readily visible areas or manual dexterity or memory is a potential concern for adherence. A caregiver may be enlisted to assist with self-applied topical therapies, with written instructions and areas of treatment outlined. Because of the lower rate of cure for topical field therapies compared to excision or Mohs the ability to follow up in clinic for skin cancer surveillance is essential when considering this modality.

Recent data from a large European multicenter randomized controlled trial of photodynamic therapy (MAL-PDT) versus topical imiquimod versus topical fluorouracil for superficial BCCs demonstrated that imiquimod was superior to MAL-PDT, and that topical 5FU was non-inferior at 12-month follow-up [18]. The average age of patients in each arm ranged from 62 to 64 years old. Cure rates at 12 months were 93 % for imiquimod (regimen was 5 days a week for 6 weeks), 91 % for fluorouracil (regimen was twice a day for 4 weeks), and 87 % for MAL-PDT (3-h incubation under occlusion ×2 treatments).

Electrodesiccation and curettage can result in 5-year cure rates of 82–94 % for BCCs; however in one large study up to 15 % of patients experienced hypertrophic scars [19, 20]. More recent data on quality-of-life outcomes of treatments for cutaneous BCC and SCC in individuals with mean age over 65 showed that patients who underwent electrodesiccation and curettage report lower quality of life compared to excision or Mohs surgery [21].

Cryotherapy monotherapy has been considered in individuals with BCC often as a treatment only when no other good choices are available. For instance, recent case reports in older individuals illustrate their potential utility [22]. However, good-quality data in superficial BCCs has been reported in randomized studies compared head to head with MALA PDT (3-h incubation up to three sessions), and found to have similar recurrence rates at 5 years (up to two treatments, each with two freeze-thaw cycles) but inferior cosmetic results [23].

Recently, retrospective data from 631 BCCs treated with superficial radiation therapy has been reported. This modality utilizes ionizing radiation, or electronic surface brachytherapy, which consists of low-energy photon X-rays. These treatments are being used increasingly by dermatologists, in conjunction with radiation oncologists. Compared to traditional radiation therapy, SRT and eSBT consist of fewer treatments and can be delivered in the outpatient setting without a linear accelerator. Aggregate data from superficial and nodular BCCs 5 years after treatment revealed a recurrence rate of 4.2 % [24]. Higher recurrence rates occurred in tumors greater than 2 cm. Cosmetic outcomes have not been addressed, particularly in head-to-head comparison with other treatment modalities. While superficial radiation therapy may be considered in individuals who cannot or will not undergo surgical treatment or topical pharmacotherapy, concerns about costs of superficial radiation therapy, risk of radiation dermatitis, and secondary cancers remain to be studied further.

One of the largest recent breakthroughs in skin cancer therapy over the past 5 years is the commercial availability of smoothened inhibitors, a targeted way to disrupt the Hedgehog signaling pathway in advanced basal cell carcinomas. In the largest multicenter clinical study to date of targeted therapy for advanced basal cell carcinoma (unresectable or metastatic), 119 patients with an average age of 62 years demonstrated a 46.4 % response rate [25] after a median of 5.5 months of vismodegib exposure. When this data was broken down by age greater or equal to 65 years versus less than or equal to 65 years [26] there was no significant difference in the overall response rate by age. There did not appear to be significant differences in frequency of side effects either. However, in those under 65 years, the percentage of individuals with grade 3 or higher side effects was 2 % in those aged 65 or less compared to 11 % in those aged 65 or greater, suggesting that the severity of side effects in adults aged 65 or older may be greater than those under 65. Future larger studies may identify covariates that might explain the increased severity in adverse events in older adults.

Cutaneous Squamous Cell Carcinoma in Older Adults

Like stage I and II BCCs, the gold standard therapy for stage I and II cutaneous squamous cell carcinoma (CSCC) continues to be excision, offering the highest cure rates [27]. In one pooled average of 12 studies ($n=1,144$) the local recurrence rate after excision was 5.4 % and in a pooled average of 10 studies ($n=1,572$) the local recurrence rate after Mohs micrographic surgery was 3.0 % [27]. For CSCCs with two or more high-risk features (such as size, depth of invasion, perineural spread, location on the lip or ear) adjuvant radiation after excision can be considered. For SCCs with perineural invasion treated with adjuvant radiotherapy, pooled local recurrence average based on five studies ($n=22$) was 18.2 %, and for SCCs without perineural invasion, pooled local recurrence average based on four studies was 11.1 % [27].

For patients with invasive CSCC who cannot tolerate surgery or decline surgery, a number of treatment options exist, although the cure rates are much lower and close follow-up monitoring for recurrence is required. For instance, in one small study of 26 patients with face and neck CSCC who had declined surgery or experienced treatment failure after surgery, photodynamic therapy with red light led to complete response rate of 77 % at 48 months [28]. Due to the small study, delineation of clinical or histologic characteristics most likely to result in cure is unclear. However, other data on photodynamic therapy indicates high recurrence rates after apparent initial response that averaged 26.4 % ($n=119$) [27]. Other treatment modalities in the literature include curettage and electrodesiccation of SCCs (generally less than 2 cm), in seven studies and variable follow-up periods, with indicated recurrence average of 1.7 % ($n=1,131$). For cryotherapy, the recurrence average was 0.8 % based on eight studies ($n=273$) for low-risk SCCs less than 2 cm [27].

For small invasive CSCCs, another modality that has seen increasing use in the older population is superficial X-ray therapy (SXRT). While the published short-term response rates are high, with only 1.8 % recurrence at 2 years and 5.8 % recurrence at 5 years for SXRT in one study with 994 SCC patients [24], issues urgently needing study include which sites are most amenable to treatment, characteristics of "low-risk" SCCs that make

SRT a good choice, cost-benefit considerations due to significant cost of SRT, optimal number of treatments, and risk of long-term secondary cancers. In one retrospective study of superficial radiation treatment for 180 large cutaneous SCCs (mean age late 60s) in Switzerland, relapse-free survival was 95 % after 1 year and 80 % after 10 years [29], with the anatomic location showing the highest relapse-free survival as around the eyes and on the cheek.

For SCC in situ (SCCIS), excision still confers the highest cure rate although topical therapies can be a good choice, with the same caveats in the elderly population as discussed above. There is level II evidence for the use of topical imiquimod (5 % daily × 16 weeks) for SCCIS, with randomized study showing resolution of 73 % of SCCIS at 9 months [12, 30]. The use of topical 5-fluorouracil (one to two times daily, up to two cycles of 4 and 6 weeks) and ALA photodynamic therapy (4-h incubation) for SCCIS is based on level 4 evidence with 12-month response rates reported at 82 % and 48 %, respectively [12, 31].

A recent retrospective case–control study of 25 cases of advanced CSCC in adults with a median age of 66 years showed that 70 % of patients with unresectable do not respond to any treatment. Only cisplatin was found to alter overall survival (OS) and progression-free survival (PFS). Neither taxane and cetuximab nor multiagent therapy improved OS or PFS. Only two patients received radiation, precluding assessment of OS and PFS.

A larger retrospective study of 61 patients (median age in the 70s) who had resected head and neck CSCC did not show any difference in overall survival between individuals receiving postsurgical adjuvant radiation versus adjuvant chemoradiation, although adjuvant chemoradiation significantly decreased the risk of recurrence or death in a multivariable analysis with a hazard ratio of 0.31 [32].

Promising lines of investigation into new treatments for unresectable or metastatic CSCC include capecitabine or immunotherapy such as PD1/PD-L1 pathway inhibitors.

Melanoma in Older Adults

A 2013 population-based study from France demonstrated differences in the epidemiology and management of melanoma in older adults, defined as 70 years or older. Elderly patients demonstrated a higher percentage of particular melanoma subtypes such as acral and lentigo maligna melanoma, melanoma of the head and neck, thicker melanomas at the time of diagnosis, and a higher percentage of ulceration [33]. The finding of thicker melanomas in older individuals is confirmed in a separate retrospective study of the National Cancer Institute's Surveillance, Epidemiology and End Results database from 2004 to 2008 in which a statistically significant increase in ulceration in older men in for cutaneous melanoma that was 2 mm or thicker [34] was found.

Regarding differences in melanoma management, older patients were more likely to have their melanomas diagnosed in the primary care setting rather than by the dermatologist in France [33]. In addition, practice gaps in older adults included a significantly lower percentage of elderly receiving adequate margins on excision, sentinel lymph node biopsy (SLNB), and adjuvant therapy [33].

Other studies have supported these findings, in particular, the lower rate of SLNB in older melanoma patients. A recent retrospective study assessed the actual reasons in 358 patients aged 65 years or older with melanoma greater than or equal to 1 mm thickness. Reasons for omission of SLNB included selective neck dissection (7 %), patient refusal (3 %), physician recommendation (4 %), and significant comorbidities (2 %) [35]. In general, SLNB in those who did undergo the procedure was successful in over 98 % of patients, with high sensitivity rate (90.5 %), and low false-negative rate (3.8 %), suggesting that age alone should not be a contraindication for SLNB in melanoma [35]. In this group, SLN status was independently associated with melanoma-specific survival. Further studies are needed to identify reasons for the practice discrepancies identified to date for melanoma detection and care, and whether there may an age bias contributing to these differences.

Targeted chemotherapies in use for melanoma patients with unresectable disease include vemurafenib, a BRAF kinase inhibitor shown in a phase 3 randomized clinical trial against dacarbazine to improve survival and disease-free survival in 675 patients with previously untreated metastatic melanoma with the BRAF V600E mutation [36] with mean age in the 50s of the study participants. More recently, additional overall response and progression-free survival were seen by combining BRAF inhibitor dabrafenib with an MEK inhibitor trametinib in a phase 3 clinical trial with average age of participants in the 50s [37].

Exciting new chemotherapies for advanced melanomas include immune checkpoint inhibitors. Ipilimumab is a drug in this class and works by blocking downregulation of cytotoxic T-lymphocyte-associated antigen 4-mediated T cell activation [38], shown in phase 3 trials in populations with mean age in the 50s to be beneficial for overall survival. Other checkpoint inhibitors block PD1/PDL1 signaling, and recent phase 3 studies of pembrolizumab (now commercially available) and nivolumab have shown overall survival benefit for stage 3 or 4 melanoma, the latter against dacarbazine in patients with mean age in the 60s in clinical trials [39, 40]. Treatment options are rapidly evolving in melanoma, an unmet area of medical need as melanoma incidence continues to rise worldwide.

References

1. Kricker A, Armstrong B, Hansen V, Watson A, Singh-Khaira G, Lecathelinais C, et al. Basal cell carcinoma and squamous cell carcinoma growth rates and determinants of size in community patients. J Am Acad Dermatol. 2014;70(3):456–64.
2. Rashtak S, Dierkhising RA, Kremers WK, Peters SG, Cassivi SD, Otley CC. Incidence and risk factors for skin cancer following lung transplantation. J Am Acad Dermatol. 2015;72(1):92–8.
3. Sekulic A, Migden MR, Oro AE, Dirix L, Lewis KD, Hainsworth JD, et al. Efficacy and safety of vismodegib in advanced basal cell carcinoma. N Engl J Med. 2012;366(23):2171–9.
4. McArthur GA, Chapman PB, Robert C, Larkin J, Haanen J, Dummer R, et al. Safety and efficacy of

vemurafenib in *BRAF*[V600E] and *BRAF*[V600K] mutation-positive melanoma (BRIM-3): extended follow-up of a phase 3, randomised, open-label study. Lancet Oncology. 2014;15(3):323–32.

5. Tumeh PC, Harview CL, Yearley JH, Shintaku IP, Taylor EJ, Robert L, et al. PD-1 blockade induces responses by inhibiting adaptive immune resistance. Nature. 2014;515(7528):568–71.

6. Petit JY, Avril MF, Margulis A, Chassagne D, Gerbaulet A, Duvillard P, et al. Evaluation of cosmetic results of a randomized trial comparing surgery and radiotherapy in the treatment of basal cell carcinoma of the face. Plast Reconstr Surg. 2000;105(7): 2544–51.

7. Smeets NW, Krekels GA, Ostertag JU, Essers BA, Dirksen CD, Nieman FH, et al. Surgical excision vs Mohs' micrographic surgery for basal-cell carcinoma of the face: randomised controlled trial. Lancet. 2004;364(9447):1766–72.

8. Rhodes LE, de Rie M, Enström Y, Groves R, Morken T, Goulden V, et al. Photodynamic therapy using topical methyl aminolevulinate vs surgery for nodular basal cell carcinoma: results of a multicenter randomized prospective trial. Arch Dermatol. 2004;140(1): 17–23.

9. Thissen MR, Nieman FH, Ideler AH, Berretty PJ, Neumann HA. Cosmetic results of cryosurgery versus surgical excision for primary uncomplicated basal cell carcinomas of the head and neck. Dermatol Surg. 2000;26(8):759–64.

10. Olsen CM, Williams PF, Whiteman DC. Turning the tide? Changes in treatment rates for keratinocytic cancers in Australia 2000-2011. J Am Acad Dermatol. 2014;7(1):21–6.

11. Love WE, Bernhard JD, Bordeaux JS. Topical imiquimod or fluorouracil therapy for basal and squamous cell carcinoma. Arch Dermatol. 2009;145(12): 1431–8.

12. Micali G, Lacarrubba F, Nasca MR, Ferraro S, Schwartz RA. Topical pharmacotherapy for skin cancer. J Am Acad Dermatol. 2014;6(e1):979.e12.

13. Beutner KR, Geisse JK, Helman D, Fox TL, Ginkel A, Owens ML. Therapeutic response of basal cell carcinoma to the immune response modifier imiquimod 5 % cream. J Am Acad Dermatol. 1999;41(6):1002–7.

14. Geisse JK, Rich P, Pandya A, Gross K, Andres K, Ginkel A, et al. Imiquimod 5% cream for the treatment of superficial basal cell carcinoma: a double-blind, randomized, vehicle-controlled study. J Am Acad Dermatol. 2002;47(3):390–8.

15. Shumack S, Robinson J, Kossard S, Golitz L, Greenway H, Schroeter A, et al. Efficacy of topical 5% imiquimod cream for the treatment of nodular basal cell carcinoma: comparison of dosing regimens. Arch Dermatol. 2002;138(9):1165–71.

16. Marks R1, Gebauer K, Shumack S, Amies M, Bryden J, Fox TL, et al. Australasian Multicentre Trial Group. Imiquimod 5 % cream in the treatment of superficial basal cell carcinoma: results of a multicenter 6-week

dose-response trial. J Am Acad Dermatol. 2001; 44(5):807–13.

17. Schulze HJ, Cribier B, Requena L, Reifenberger J, Ferrándiz C, Garcia Diez A, et al. Imiquimod 5% cream for the treatment of superficial basal cell carcinoma: results from a randomized vehicle-controlled phase III study in Europe. Br J Dermatol. 2005; 152(5):939–47.

18. Arits AH, Mosterd K, Essers BA, Spoorenberg E, Sommer A, De Rooij MJ, et al. Photodynamic therapy versus topical imiquimod versus topical fluorouracil for treatment of superficial basal-cell carcinoma: a single blind, non-inferiority, randomized controlled trial. Lancet Oncology. 2013;14(7):647–54.

19. Kopf AW, Bart RS, Schrager D. Curettage-electrodessication treatment of basal cell carcinomas. Arch Dermatol. 1977;113:439–43.

20. Hansen TJ, Anderson BE. Electrodessication and curettage for low-risk cutaneous malignancies of the head and neck. Oper Tech Otolaryngol-Head Neck Surg. 2013;24(1):55.

21. Chren M, Sahay AP, Bertenthal DS, Sen S, Landefeld CS. Quality of life outcomes of treatments for cutaneous basal cell carcinoma and squamous cell carcinoma. J Investig Dermatol. 2007;6:1351–7.

22. Chiriac A, Mihaila D, Foia L, Solovan C. Basal cell carcinomas in elderly patients treated by cryotherapy. Clin Interv Aging. 2013;8:341–4.

23. Basset-Seguin N, Ibbotson SH, Emtestam L, Tarstedt M, Morton C, Maroti M, et al. Topical methyl aminolevulinate photodynamic therapy versus cryotherapy for superficial basal cell carcinoma: a 5 year randomized trial. Eur J Dermatol. 2008;18(5): 547–53.

24. Cognetta AB, Howard BM, Heaton HP, Stoddard ER, Hong HG, Green WH. Superficial x-ray in the treatment of basal and squamous cell carcinomas: a viable option in select patients. J Am Acad Dermatol. 2012;67(6):1235–41.

25. Chang AL, Solomon JA, Hainsworth JD, Goldberg L, McKenna E, Day B, et al. Expanded access study of advanced basal cell carcinoma patients treated with the Hedgehog pathway inhibitor, vismodegib. J Am Acad Dermatol. 2014;70(1):60–9.

26. Chang ALS, Lewis K, Arron ST, Migden M, Solomon J, et al. (2015) Safety and efficacy of vismodegib in elderly patients: analysis of the ERIVANCE BCC and expanded access studies. J Am Acad Dermatol. (in press)

27. Lansbury L, Bath-Hextall F, Perkins W, Stanton W, Leonardi-Bee J. Interventions for non-metastatic squamous cell carcinoma of the skin: systematic review and pooled analysis of observational studies. BMJ. 2013;347:f6153.

28. Wenig BL, Kurtzman DM, Grossweiner LI, Mafee MF, Harris DM, Lobraico RV, et al. Photodynamic therapy in the treatment of squamous cell carcinoma of the head and neck. Arch Otolaryngol Head Neck Surg. 1990;116(11):1267–70.

29. Barysch MJ, Eggmann N, Beyeler M, Panizzon RG, Seifert B, Dummer R. Long-term recurrence rate of large and difficult to treat cutaneous squamous cell carcinomas after superficial radiotherapy. Dermatology. 2012;224(1):59–65.

30. Patel GK, Goodwin R, Chawla M, Laidler P, Price PE, Finlay AY, et al. Imiquimod 5% cream monotherapy for cutaneous squamous cell carcinoma in situ (Bowen's disease): a randomized, double blind, placebo-controlled trial. J Am Acad Dermatol. 2006;54:1025–32.

31. Salim A, Leman JA, McColl JH, Chapman R, Morton CA. Randomized comparison of photodynamic therapy with topical 5-fluorouracil in Bowen's disease. Br J Dermatol. 2003;148:539–43.

32. Tanvetyanon T, Padhya T, McCaffrey J, Kish JA, Deconti RC, Trotti A, et al. Postoperative concurrent chemotherapy and radiotherapy for high-risk cutaneous squamous cell carcinoma of the head and neck. Head Neck. 2014 Mar 12. doi:10.1002/hed.23684. [Epub ahead of print]

33. Ciocan D, Barbe C, Aubin F, Granel-Brocard F, Lipsker D, Velten M, et al. Distinctive features of melanoma and its management in elderly patients. JAMA Dermatol. 2013;149(10):1150–7.

34. Richardson BS, Anderson WF, Barnholtz-Sloan JS, Tucker MA, Gerstenblith MR. The age-specific effect modification of male sex for ulcerated cutaneous melanoma. JAMA Dermatol. 2014;150(5):522–5.

35. Grotz TE, Puig CA, Perkins S, Ballman K, Hieken TJ. Management of regional lymph nodes in the elderly melanoma patient: patient selection, accuracy and prognostic implications. Eur J Surg Oncol. 2014;0748–83.

36. Chapman PB, Hauschild A, Robert C, Haanen JB, Ascierto P, Larkin J, et al. Improved survival with vemburafenib in melanoma with BRAF V600E mutation. NEJM. 2011;364:2507–16.

37. Long GV, Stoyakovskiy H, Gogas E, Levchenko E, de Braud F, Larkin J, et al. Combined BRAF and MEK inhibition versus BRAF inhibition alone in melanoma. NEJM. 2014;37:1877–88.

38. Hodi FS, O'Day SJ, McDermott DF, Weber RW, Sosman JA, Haanen JB, et al. Improved survival with ipilimumab in patients with metastatic melanoma. NEJM. 2010;363(8):711–23.

39. Hamid O, Robert C, Daud A, Hodi FS, Hwu WJ, Kefford R, et al. Safety and tumor responses with lambrolizumab (anti-PD-1) in melanoma. N Engl J Med. 2013;369(2):134–44.

40. Robert C, Long GV, Brady B, Dutriaux C, Maio M, Mortier L, et al. Nivolumab in previously untreated melanoma without BRAF mutation. NEJM. 2015;372:320–30.

Index

© Springer International Publishing Switzerland 2015
A.L.S. Chang (ed.), *Advances in Geriatric Dermatology*, DOI 10.1007/978-3-319-18380-0